Management of Atrial Fibrillation

OXFORD CARDIOLOGY LIBRARY

Management of Atrial Fibrillation

A Practical Approach

Edited by

Mohammad Shenasa MD

Attending Physician
Department of Cardiovascular Services
O'Connor Hospital;
Heart & Rhythm Medical Group
San Jose, CA, USA

A. John Camm MD

Professor of Clinical Cardiology
Department of Clinical Sciences
St George's and University of London
London, UK

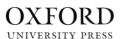

OXFORD
UNIVERSITY PRESS

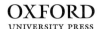

Great Clarendon Street, Oxford, OX2 6DP,
United Kingdom

Oxford University Press is a department of the University of Oxford.
It furthers the University's objective of excellence in research, scholarship,
and education by publishing worldwide. Oxford is a registered trade mark of
Oxford University Press in the UK and in certain other countries

Published in the United States of America by Oxford University Press 198
Madison Avenue, New York, NY 10016, United States of America

British Library Cataloguing in Publication Data
Data available

Library of Congress Control Number: 2014947265

ISBN 978–0–19–968631–5

Printed in Great Britain by
Ashford Colour Press Ltd, Gosport, Hampshire

To our patients who taught us the most.
To our colleagues who took care of our patients.
To our families for their infinite support and love.

Mohammad Shenasa
A. John Camm

Contents

Contributors

A. John Camm MD

Professor of Clinical Cardiology
Clinical Sciences
St George's University of London
London, UK

Anne B. Curtis MD

UB Distinguished Professor
Charles and Mary Bauer Professor
and Chair
Department of Medicine
University at Buffalo
Buffalo, NY, USA

Harry J.G.M. Crijns

Chair, Department of Cardiology
University Hospital Maastricht
Maastricht University Medical Center
The Netherlands

Christos Dresios MD

University of Birmingham Centre for
Cardiovascular Sciences
City Hospital
Birmingham, UK

Bernard J. Gersh MD

Professor of Medicine
Mayo Clinic College of Medicine
Rochester, MN, USA

Gregory Y.H. Lip MD

Professor of Cardiovascular Medicine
University of Birmingham Centre for
Cardiovascular Sciences
City Hospital
Birmingham, UK

Christopher McLeod MD

Assistant Professor of Medicine
Mayo Clinic College of Medicine
Rochester, MN, USA

L. Brent Mitchell MD

Professor of Medicine
Libin Cardiovascular Institute of Alberta
Alberta Health Services and University
of Calgary
Alberta, Canada

Bart A. Mulder MD

University Medical Center
Groningen
Hanzeplein, The Netherlands

Cevher Ozcan MD

Assistant Professor
Department of Medicine
University at Buffalo
Buffalo, NY, USA

Shahrzad Rouhani

Heart and Rhythm Medical Group
San Jose, CA, USA

James A. Reiffel MD

Professor of Medicine (at CUMC)
Columbia University
Attending Physician and co-Director
Electrocardiography Laboratory
The New York Presbyterian Hospital
New York, NY, USA

Irene Savelieva MD

Lecturer in Clinical Cardiology
Division of Clinical Sciences
Cardiology Section
St George's University of London
London, UK

Hossein Shenasa MD

Attending Physician
Department of Cardiovascular Services
O'Connor Hospital
San Jose, CA, USA
California Heart & Rhythm Medical
Group
San Jose, CA, USA

Mohammad Shenasa MD

Attending Physician
Department of Cardiovascular Services
O'Connor Hospital, San Jose
California Heart & Rhythm Medical Group
San Jose, CA, USA

Isabelle C. Van Gelder MD

Professor of Cardiology
Director of Electrophysiology
University Medical Center Groningen
Hanzeplein, The Netherlands

Preface

The last two decades we have witnessed significant progress in the understanding of atrial fibrillation, from its pathophysiology to its complex and diverse etiologies and relation to most devastating complication, stroke. Despite several recent breakthroughs on novel oral anticoagulation, antiarrhythmic agents and interventional procedures, we are still losing the battle or the management remains at least unsatisfactory. This in part may be due to the evolving nature of this rhythm disorder and the fact all atrial fibrillations are not the same, thus we are not dealing with the same entity.

Despite many guidelines and consensus from many medical societies as well as several large texts on the subject we feel that there exists a gap between academic centers and practitioners who indeed see 80% of patients with AF.

This short text is therefore designed to provide the most recent evidence-based information and how to deal with patients with Atrial Fibrillation. The target audiences of this book are primary physicians, Emergency room doctors, hospitalists, internists, and generally cardiologists who care after the majority of these patients.

We would like to thank our colleagues who provided their up to date evidence-based manuscripts.

Finally we are thankful to the Oxford University Press staff, namely Helen Liepman, James Oates, and Emily Richardson, for their excellent support in completing this volume.

The Editors:
Mohammad Shenasa & A. John Camm

Foreword

Atrial fibrillation is an arrhythmia that is easy to recognize but difficult to treat. Not having the right focus may be deleterious for patients suffering from this arrhythmia. Over the past decades an increasing number of studies have been performed and several guidelines have been issued to improve management of atrial fibrillation. Initially, the main focus of management was on controlling the rhythm by cardioversion and antiarrhythmic drugs, shifting to antithrombotic treatment in the early nineties of the previous century. However, patients with atrial fibrillation are not only threatened by stroke but even more by heart failure and cardiovascular death. Therefore, the large rhythm versus rate control studies—including for instance AFFIRM, AF-CHF and ATHENA—appropriately used major adverse cardiovascular and cerebrovascular events as an endpoint. As a consequence, we nowadays know very well that upstream therapy—which is nothing more and nothing less than adequately and aggressively treating the underlying cardiovascular diseases associated with atrial fibrillation—is of utmost importance to prevent further harm. Eventually, all this helped to reduce morbidity and mortality rates in patients with atrial fibrillation. Notwithstanding the above, daily management of atrial fibrillation remains a challenge. In addition, early identification of high risk patients—even going beyond the well-known clinical prediction schemes of CHA2DS2-VASc and HAS-BLED—and early personalized treatment to prevent atrial fibrillation progression are new dots on the management horizon.

In this book Drs. Shenasa and Camm provide us not only with a concise and practical account on daily management of atrial fibrillation but also new cutting edge clinical ideas to enhance personalized treatment for individual patients. To prepare this volume they brought together an excellent group of scientists and clinicians who share their knowledge and latest insights. The book presents extremely useful schemes and summary boxes to direct daily patient care. It contains a series of chapters providing solid guidance on—among others—the work-up of first detected atrial fibrillation, the complexity of antiarrhythmic therapy and appropriateness of antithrombotic therapy, or on when to refer a patient for an arrhythmia intervention. Reading on latest insights may trigger new personal clinical views and research ideas. I am fully confident that this book will prove to be valuable to specialists, trainees and researchers in cardiology, internal medicine, neurology, geriatric medicine as well as family practice. As such, it will certainly contribute to improved care for patients with atrial fibrillation.

Harry J.G.M. Crijns
Chair, Department of Cardiology
University Hospital Maastricht
Maastricht University Medical Center
The Netherlands

Abbreviations

AAD	antiarrhythmic drugs
AF	atrial fibrillation
AFNET	German Competence Network on Atrial Fibrillation
ACC	American College of Cardiology
ACE	angiotensin-converting enzyme
ACS	acute coronary syndromes
AF	atrial fibrillation
AHA	American Heart Association
aPTT	activated partial thromboplastin time
ARB	angiotensin receptor blocker
ASA	acetylsalicylic acid
AV	atrioventricular
AVRT	atrioventricular re-entrant tachycardia
BNP	B-type natriuretic peptide
BP	blood pressure
bpm	beats per minute
CABG	coronary artery bypass graft
CAD	coronary artery disease
COPD	chronic obstructive pulmonary disease
CrCl	creatinine clearance
CRP	C-reactive protein
CRT	cardiac resynchronization therapy
CYP	cytochrome
ECG	electrocardiogram
ECT	clotting time
EHRA	European Heart Rhythm Association
EMA	European Medicines Agency
ESC	European Society of Cardiology
FDA	Food and Drug Administration
FFP	fresh frozen plasma
GI	gastrointestinal
HAS-BLED	hypertension, abnormal renal/liver function, stroke, bleeding history or bleeding tendency, labile INR, elderly, drugs/alcohol use
HCM	hypertrophic cardiomyopathy

HF	heart failure
HRS	Heart Rhythm Society
ICD	implantable cardioverter defibrillator
INR	international normalized ratio
LAA	left atrial appendage
LMWH	low-molecular-weight heparin
LV	left ventricular
LVH	left ventricular hypertrophy
MI	myocardial infarction
MRI	magnetic resonance imaging
NHS	National Health Service
NOAC	new oral anticoagulant agent
NSAID	non-steroidal anti-inflammatory drug
NYHA	New York Heart Association
OAC	oral anticoagulant
PAD	peripheral arterial disease
PAF	paroxysmal atrial fibrillation
PCI	percutaneous coronary intervention
P-gp	P-glycoprotein
PT	prothrombin time
PVD	peripheral vascular disease
SHD	structural heart diseases
SVT	supraventricular tachycardia
TCT	thrombin clotting time
TIA	transient ischaemic attack
TOE	transoesophageal echocardiogram
TSH	thyroid stimulating hormone
TT	triple therapy
TTR	time in therapeutic range
UFH	unfractionated heparin
VF	ventricular fibrillation
VHD	valvular heart disease
VKA	vitamin K antagonist
VT	ventricular tachycardia

Chapter 1

The epidemiology of atrial fibrillation

Christopher McLeod and Bernard J. Gersh

Key points

- Atrial fibrillation (AF) is the most common sustained rhythm abnormality, and is more common in the older patient—occurring in over 10% of patients over the age of 80.
- It is most commonly associated with adjunctive cardiac disease.
- It is associated with around 15% of all strokes.
- The number of people with AF will likely increase several-fold by 2050.
- Most of the money spent on AF is related to hospitalizations.

1.1 Introduction to the epidemiology of atrial fibrillation

Atrial fibrillation (AF) is the most common sustained rhythm abnormality and presents as paroxysmal and persistent forms. It is also one of the most common cardiovascular diseases and a major cause of stroke in developed countries, constituting a significant public health problem. This arrhythmia does occur in isolation, yet it is more commonly seen in conjunction with cardiovascular disease, hypertension, diabetes, sleep apnoea, and obesity. In association with these co-morbidities, the presence of AF is associated with an increase in mortality, but moreover distinctly affects quality of life and leads to numerous emergency room visits and hospitalizations. The prevalence of AF is expected to rise considerably as the population ages. Current estimates suggest that this condition accounts for 1% of the National Health Service (NHS) budget in the United Kingdom and US$16–26 billion of annual Medicare expenditure in the United States.

1.2 Risk factors for the development of atrial fibrillation

The older male Caucasian in a low socioeconomic group presents the highest risk demographic profile for the development of AF. Adverse lifestyle factors include smoking, significant alcohol intake, and obesity, while cardiovascular diseases such as hypertension, left ventricular hypertrophy, coronary disease, and left atrial enlargement all increase the likelihood for the development of AF. In addition, other co-morbidities such as diabetes, pulmonary disease, hypothyroidism, and obstructive sleep apnoea (OSA) are all major risk factors for the development of AF. Cardiothoracic surgery, including coronary bypass surgery, is a substantial risk factor for the development of AF in the postoperative period.

1.3 **Incidence, prevalence, and lifetime risk**

The incidence of AF increases with age, remaining uncommon before the age of 70 years, but rising exponentially at this point. It is also more commonly seen in males across all age groups, and in those with cardiovascular disease. Black people have less than half the age-adjusted risk for developing AF compared with white people and lone AF (without structural heart disease) occurs in less than a quarter of cases. Data from the Framingham and Rotterdam studies suggest the lifetime risk of any single person developing AF is around one in four. It is also important to recognize that subclinical AF is common, and not infrequently presents as stroke. Recent data from pacemaker recordings in patients without a prior diagnosis of AF has unveiled a substantial body of patients with this subclinical 'cryptogenic' AF, suggesting that the incidence and prevalence is much higher.

1.4 **Primary care visits**

Data from large UK and Dutch studies indicate that AF is a presenting diagnosis in less than 1% of patients below the age of 40, yet it occurs in around 10% of patients over the age of 80 in the primary care setting. These rates are continuing to rise, in parallel to the overall prevalence.

1.5 **Hospitalizations**

Across most developed countries, AF accounts for around 10–20 per 10,000 hospital admissions as the primary diagnosis. If one looks specifically at patients over the age of 65, the admission rates are up to ten fold higher, and this has consistently risen over the last two decades. The most common co-morbidities are heart failure and coronary disease.

1.6 **Health outcomes**

1.6.1 **Prognosis**

The development of AF is associated with around a 1.5–2-fold increase in cardiovascular and all-cause mortality. Women are found to be consistently at higher risk, with up to a fivefold increased risk of a cardiovascular event when AF is concomitantly diagnosed.

1.6.2 **Stroke and AF**

AF is a major independent risk factor for stroke, and increases the risk by three- to fivefold. Strokes associated with AF are also more severe, resulting in a higher likelihood of dying, but also longer hospital stays, more neurological damage, and greater disability.

1.6.3 **Heart failure and AF**

Epidemiological association studies of heart failure and AF have revealed an incestuous relationship, with heart failure contributing to the development of AF and AF contributing to the development of heart failure. Over a third of patients with a diagnosis of heart failure will develop AF at some stage, and the presence of AF alone increases the risk of heart failure by around four- to sixfold, with women again being at higher risk.

1.6.4 **Acute coronary syndromes and AF**

There is also an intimate relationship between acute coronary syndromes (ACS) and AF with up to a fifth of patients with an ACS developing AF during their hospitalization. This development of AF is consequently associated with an increase in acute and long-term mortality and this is probably a manifestation of left ventricular dysfunction with increased filling pressures. This is more likely to occur in the older patient with a faster heart rate at admission and those with concomitant heart failure.

1.6.5 **AF and hypertension**

Hypertension is probably the largest single contributor to the development of AF in a population. The presence of hypertension alone increases the risk of developing AF by 70–80% in men and women, and is the likely cause of at least a fifth of the AF in the developed world.

1.6.6 **AF and OSA**

Although AF and OSA share similar risk factors, there is nevertheless around a 3.5-fold increased risk for the development of AF if OSA is present. There is also emerging data that effective treatment of OSA lowers this risk, and also lowers the risk of recurrence of AF after direct-current cardioversion and ablation for AF.

1.6.7 **AF and obesity**

A linear association between increasing body mass index (BMI) and the development of AF has been well defined. Obese patients (BMI > 30) experience approximately a 5% increase in their risk of developing AF for every unit of increase in their BMI. In the United States, it is also postulated that the majority (60%) of the estimated increase in AF incidence is potentially attributable to the obesity epidemic itself.

1.7 **Economic burden of AF**

Hospitalization costs account for almost half of the money spent either directly or indirectly on AF as the primary diagnosis. This condition accounts for 1% of the NHS budget in the United Kingdom and US$16–26 billion of annual US Medicare expenses. Across the developed world this can amount to as high as 2.5% of the national healthcare expenditure. As addressed in this chapter, AF complicates hospitalizations for heart failure, ACS, stroke, and so on, therefore prolonging inpatient stays and increasing cost further. There has also been a dramatic rise in the incidence of AF in nursing homes, thereby complicating chronic therapy and increasing cost.

1.8 **Future burden of AF**

All current estimates suggest that the burden of AF will continue to increase over the next few decades, with estimates varying between a three- to sevenfold increase in the number of patients with AF by the year 2050. In addition, it appears that most of these patients will be older, and it is likely that around 50% will be over the age of 80 years.

1.9 **Conclusion to the epidemiology of AF**

The epidemiology of AF identifies that this disease process is intimately linked with other cardiovascular co-morbidities. In addition, these studies hallmark that the incidence and prevalence is growing rapidly as the developed world struggles to master an obesity epidemic and as their populations live longer. Therapies for AF will therefore also need to target co-morbid conditions if we are to successfully manage this arrhythmia.

Key reading

Crenshaw BS, Ward SR, Granger CB, Stebbins AL, Topol EJ, Califf RM. Atrial fibrillation in the setting of acute myocardial infarction: the GUSTO-I experience. Global Utilization of Streptokinase and TPA for Occluded Coronary Arteries. *J Am Coll Cardiol* 1997; 30(2): 406–13.

Gami AS, Hodge DO, Herges RM, Olson EJ, Nykodym J, Kara T, et al. Obstructive sleep apnea, obesity, and the risk of incident atrial fibrillation. *J Am Coll Cardiol* 2007; 49(5): 565–71.

Gami AS, Pressman G, Caples SM, Kanagala R, Gard JJ, Davison DE, et al. Association of atrial fibrillation and obstructive sleep apnea. *Circulation* 2004; 110(4): 364–7.

Go AS, Hylek EM, Phillips KA, Chang Y, Henault LE, Selby JV, et al. Prevalence of diagnosed atrial fibrillation in adults: national implications for rhythm management and stroke prevention: the AnTicoagulation and Risk Factors in Atrial Fibrillation (ATRIA) Study. *JAMA* 2001; 285(18): 2370–5.

Heeringa J, van der Kuip DA, Hofman A, Kors JA, van Herpen G, Stricker BH, et al. Prevalence, incidence and lifetime risk of atrial fibrillation: the Rotterdam study. *Eur Heart J* 2006; 27(8): 949–53.

Hill JD, Mottram EM, Killeen PD. Study of the prevalence of atrial fibrillation in general practice patients over 65 years of age. *J R Coll Gen Pract* 1987; 37(297): 172–3.

Huxley RR, Lopez FL, Folsom AR, Agarwal SK, Loehr LR, Soliman EZ, et al. Absolute and attributable risks of atrial fibrillation in relation to optimal and borderline risk factors: the Atherosclerosis Risk in Communities (ARIC) study. *Circulation* 2011; 123(14): 1501–8.

Kim MH, Johnston SS, Chu BC, Dalal MR, Schulman KL. Estimation of total incremental health care costs in patients with atrial fibrillation in the United States. *Circ Cardiovasc Qual Outcomes* 2011; 4(3): 313–20.

Lloyd-Jones DM, Wang TJ, Leip EP, Larson MG, Levy D, Vasan RS, et al. Lifetime risk for development of atrial fibrillation: the Framingham Heart Study. *Circulation* 2004; 110(9): 1042–6.

Miyasaka Y, Barnes ME, Gersh BJ, Cha SS, Bailey KR, Abhayaratna W, et al. Incidence and mortality risk of congestive heart failure in atrial fibrillation patients: a community-based study over two decades. *Eur Heart J* 2006; 27(8): 936–41.

Miyasaka Y, Barnes ME, Gersh BJ, Cha SS, Bailey KR, Abhayaratna WP, et al. Secular trends in incidence of atrial fibrillation in Olmsted County, Minnesota, 1980 to 2000, and implications on the projections for future prevalence. *Circulation* 2006; 114(2): 119–25.

Naccarelli GV, Varker H, Lin J, Schulman KL. Increasing prevalence of atrial fibrillation and flutter in the United States. *Am J Cardiol* 2009; 104(11): 1534–9.

Schmitt J, Duray G, Gersh BJ, Hohnloser SH. Atrial fibrillation in acute myocardial infarction: a systematic review of the incidence, clinical features and prognostic implications. *Eur Heart J* 2009; 30(9): 1038–45.

Schoonderwoerd BA, Smit MD, Pen L, Van Gelder IC. New risk factors for atrial fibrillation: causes of 'not-so-lone atrial fibrillation'. *Europace* 2008; 10(6): 668–73.

Stewart S, MacIntyre K, MacLeod MM, Bailey AE, Capewell S, McMurray JJ. Trends in hospital activity, morbidity and case fatality related to atrial fibrillation in Scotland, 1986–1996. *Eur Heart J* 2001; 22(8): 69–701.

Stewart S, Murphy NF, Walker A, McGuire A, McMurray JJ. Cost of an emerging epidemic: an economic analysis of atrial fibrillation in the UK. *Heart* 2004; 90(3): 286–92.

Wattigney WA, Mensah GA, Croft JB Increasing trends in hospitalization for atrial fibrillation in the United States, 1985 through 1999: implications for primary prevention. *Circulation* 2003; 108(6): 711–16.

Wyse DG., Waldo AL, DiMarco JP, Domanski MJ, Rosenberg Y, Schron EB, et al. A comparison of rate control and rhythm control in patients with atrial fibrillation. *N Engl J Med* 2002; 347(23): 1825–33.

Chapter 2

What should be done when atrial fibrillation first presents

James A. Reiffel

Key points

- The first step in the encounter with new-onset atrial fibrillation (AF) is to determine whether immediate/urgent cardioversion is required. Significant symptoms or other evidence for notable ischaemia or haemodynamic instability will necessitate this action, as may pre-excitation with rapid antegrade conduction.

- The next step in the first encounter includes assessing the patient regarding: hints of prior episodes; possible precipitants; conditions that indicate initiation of anticoagulation; conditions that would indicate or preclude specific additional therapeutic interventions, including antiarrhythmic drugs and more; followed by or performed simultaneously with the initiation of rate control and anticoagulation (in most patients).

- If the AF was not immediately cardioverted and has not stopped spontaneously, the next step is to decide whether early non-urgent cardioversion is appropriate, and if so, whether to perform it electrically or pharmacologically. In most patients antiarrhythmic drug initiation is not indicated with the first AF episode.

- Subsequent management considerations at the first encounter include whether to schedule elective deferred cardioversion and scheduling of any additional tests required to detect and quantify important underlying disorders that may influence long-term management decisions.

- The site of the first encounter will determine additional important considerations. If it is in the emergency department, should the patient be admitted to the hospital or can he/she be safely managed as an out-patient? Ischaemia, heart failure, or an indication for continuous electrocardiogram monitoring during the first days of therapy are common indications for hospitalization. If the first encounter is in the clinic/office setting, a decision will have to be made concerning initiating evaluation and therapy as an out-patient versus an unstable state that mandates hospital referral. Finally, for the asymptomatic patient in whom AF is detected incidentally, hospitalization is not required and rhythm control may not be needed—though rate control to prevent tachycardic cardiomyopathy and anticoagulation considerations remain essential.

2.1 **Introduction to what should be done when atrial fibrillation first presents**

Current estimates suggest that over 6 million patients in the United States have atrial fibrillation (AF) and that these numbers will more than double by 2050. Worldwide these numbers are dramatically higher. And, for each of these patients, there was a first episode of AF.

When AF first presents, most often it does so with one or more symptomatic manifestations; however, it may be detected incidentally at a visit for some other clinical purpose or upon interrogation of some implanted device. The distinction between a symptomatic and an asymptomatic presentation is important because the presentation dictates much of what is done at the initial presentation, aside from the considerations of anticoagulation and rate control.

As established in the consensus statement recommending a personalized approach to the patient with AF (developed by an international group of experts at a joint meeting of the German Competence Atrial Fibrillation Network (AFNET) and the European Heart Rhythm Association (EHRA) with the support of the European Society of Cardiology (ESC) in January 2013, publication pending), a series of five steps is recommended as the considered approach when encountering a patient first presenting with AF.

2.2 **The symptomatic patient**

The care of the new-onset AF patient will depend upon how, where, and when the patient presents, his or her medical history and current medication regimen, and the presence or absence of an identifiable precipitant (see Figure 2.1).

How the patient presents is of vital importance since ischaemic and/or haemodynamic distress may be life-threatening and will require an immediate intervention whereas less dramatic symptomatology allows for a more systematic approach to evaluation and treatment. Accordingly, the first step of the five-step approach is to determine whether the

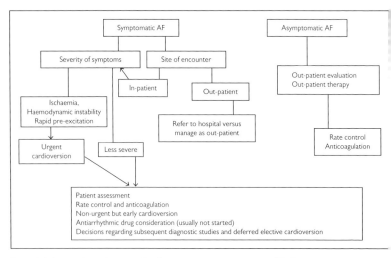

Figure 2.1 Steps and considerations when first encountering new-onset atrial fibrillation.

restoration of sinus rhythm is urgent or whether this immediate response is neither necessary nor warranted.

2.2.1 Necessity for urgent cardioversion

Ischaemic symptoms, especially if unresponsive to rapid rate-control with an intravenous drug (assuming such therapy is not precluded by hypotension) should lead to immediate pursuit of cardioversion. Ischaemia may be clear-cut by the nature of the discomfort or less certain if the patient's complaint differs from that of classic angina. The presence of either an acute injury current or significant ST depression on the electrocardiogram (ECG) should aid in this assessment. Nonetheless, because ST segment depression may be the result of underlying chronic conditions including but not limited to left ventricular hypertrophy with repolarization abnormalities, left bundle branch block, digitalis, and more, an old ECG, if available, may be of immeasurable assistance.

Significant haemodynamic instability by symptoms or physical examination (e.g. hypotension, congestive failure) also requires an immediate attempt at restoration of sinus rhythm (especially if unrelated to a rapid rate or if hypotension precludes an intravenous rate-control drug). Such instability may be exceedingly likely to occur in the presence of a hypertrophic cardiomyopathy. If possible, the caregiver should attempt to determine whether the AF is the cause of the instability, as when the rate is quite rapid, or is an associated consequence of the severe underlying cardiac disorder. For the latter, cardioversion may not provide substantial relief and, additionally, sinus rhythm is less likely to be held. Relatedly, the patient with new-onset AF is often concerned and anxious. Often a high level of sympathetic tone is accordingly present. Catecholamines can enhance the persistence and refractoriness of the arrhythmia. Hence, an additional initial step for all patients at first encounter is to comfort and reassure them to the extent possible.

A third circumstance requiring immediate intervention is pre-excitation with rapid ventricular rates. Specifically, pre-excitation with AF conducted rapidly in the antegrade direction over the bypass tract carries a significant risk of AF directly inducing ventricular fibrillation. Urgent treatment can be life-saving. Depending upon the haemodynamic instability this may require immediate cardioversion or may allow time to rapidly initiate the infusion of an intravenous antiarrhythmic agent to suppress conduction over the bypass tract and/or to rapidly induce restoration of sinus rhythm. Additionally, in this circumstance, digitalis and intravenous calcium channel blockers must be avoided as they can facilitate conduction over the bypass tract and increase the risk of VF and/or haemodynamic worsening.

Assuming immediate cardioversion has been successful or is deemed unnecessary, the second step in addressing the new-onset AF patient is to perform an initial phase of further patient assessment as well as to correct any identified reversible precipitants of or contributors to the development and continuation of AF and any that may impede further therapy.

2.2.2 Patient assessment—initial phase

An important aspect of the initial history taken from the patient is to determine whether, in fact, the current AF event is the first one the patient has experienced. Prior events including their frequency and duration will determine the need for or preferably avoidance of the initiation of antiarrhythmic therapy at this visit. Thus, the history should encompass questions regarding any prior symptoms resembling those present with this episode though they did not lead to a medical visit or were not captured by a simultaneous ECG. Most guidelines since those published jointly by the American College of Cardiology, the American Heart Association, the European Society of Cardiology, and the Heart Rhythm Society in 2001 with periodic updates thereafter recommend that chronic antiarrhythmic drugs (AADs) not be initiated for the first episode of AF. Rather, the timing and pattern of any future recurrence(s) should be determined. AADs would only carry risk without benefit if AF were not to be recurrent. And, infrequent tolerated recurrences may be treated with intermittent as-needed cardioversion (pharmacological or electrical) in preference to the burden of daily AADs. However, it may be appropriate to begin an AAD if recurrences seem likely to recur frequently due to the underlying medical circumstances and/or are felt likely to again be associated with life-threatening characteristics.

Additional important factors to determine at this point include an assessment as to the patient's reliability with respect to: accurately detecting the onset of AF; what the patient's compliance with medication regimens has been; whether there are co-morbid disorders that could affect anticoagulation and antiarrhythmic treatment decisions and choices; whether there is any evidence that indicates underlying sinus node or conduction system disease; whether there are any identifiable precipitants of the episode (Box 2.1); and whether there exist any reasons to avoid anticoagulation.

Uncertainty about the patient's ability to rapidly detect the onset of AF will preclude the use of an as-needed pharmacological (or electrical) cardioversion approach unless the patient is chronically anticoagulated. Poor medication compliance can affect the choice of an anticoagulant agent as well as considerations regarding future AAD and/or ablation options. Co-morbid conditions (Box 2.2) will affect anticoagulation necessity as they contribute to the determination of thromboembolic risk (CHADS$_2$ or CHA$_2$DS$_2$-VASc score). They will also affect AAD choices since AAD options are determined by the absence versus presence and severity of structural heart disease. Sinus node dysfunction and conduction disorders may indicate the risk of marked bradycardia upon termination of the AF episode and should lead to continuous electrocardiographic monitoring through the restitution of sinus rhythm. Detection of acute precipitants of the AF event (Box 2.1) is critical as their

---

Box 2.1 Common acute precipitants of new-onset AF

- Acute parasympathetic system (vagal) activation (including the period following strenuous activity).
- Alcohol.
- Catecholamines or other stimulants:
  - Caffeine (inconsistent opinions)
  - Cocaine, other 'recreational drugs', over-the-counter agents
  - Phaeochromocytoma (rare)
  - Secondary sympathetic activation (e.g. bleeding, etc.).
- Acute medical illness:
  - Pulmonary (pneumonia, bronchospasm, pulmonary emboli)
  - Heart failure
  - Ischaemia, myocarditis, pericarditis, cardiothoracic surgery
  - Other intrathoracic inflammatory conditions
  - Other supraventricular tachyarrhythmias
  - Metabolic (e.g. hypomagnesaemia, acid–base disorder)
  - Thyrotoxicosis (less common as a precipitant: hypothyroidism).
- Other (fever, dehydration, anaemia, and other conditions that might result in sympathetic system activation).

Box 2.2 Co-morbid conditions

Factors not identified in steps one through four including: non-acute underlying precipitants that might influence the future course of and risk for recurrent AF, non-acute conditions that affect the therapy employed, and thromboembolic risk markers:

- Hypertension
- Diabetes mellitus
- Prior stroke, transient ischaemic attack, or systemic embolus
- Sleep apnoea
- Chronic pulmonary disorders
- Intermittent pre-excitation
- Bradycardia-tachycardia syndrome
- Obesity
- Cardiomyopathy (infiltrative, etc.)
- Genetic pattern that promotes AF (elective rather than standard at the present time)
- Excessive sports (during and after).

nature may relate to the anticipated duration of the event as well as to the likelihood of recurrence if they are not corrected or avoided. Finally, since anticoagulation should be considered for all patients with AF, any contraindication, such as active bleeding, must also be determined at this point in the patient's evaluation.

Additionally, during this second stage in approaching the new-onset AF patient, specific initial laboratory studies are indicated. They may relate to precipitating contributors and/or to acute management decisions, and include:

- Haematological: CBC, electrolytes, mg, renal and hepatic function, thyroid function. (It seems increasing likely that biomarkers such as BNP, C-reactive protein, and others may be added to this early assessment if/when they are shown to affect initial management.)

- Electrocardiogram: the ECG needs to be examined for conditions beyond the rhythm diagnosis, including conduction status, repolarization duration, evidence for ischaemia, evidence for underlying structural disease, and evidence for primary electrical disorders such as Brugada pattern or pre-excitation.

- Transthoracic echocardiogram: information concerning left atrial size and function, valvular disorders, and left ventricular anatomy and function will relate to the cause of AF, risks from AF, recurrence of AF, prognosis, and therapy decisions. However, transthoracic echocardiography is not sufficiently accurate to use for detection of atrial clot.

- Chest X-ray (additional radiographic studies only if clinically indicated).

- Specifically noted in the AFNET/EHRA consensus document, there are tests which *should not* be routinely employed for AF evaluation: coronary angiography (invasive or via computed tomography scan), magnetic resonance imaging, cardiac catheterization. Infrequently they may be necessary in selected patients depending upon presentation and underlying conditions.

2.2.3 Rate control and anticoagulation

The following third step in approaching the patient with new-onset AF includes rate control and decisions regarding anticoagulation initiation.

2.2.3.1 *Rate control*

If the patient has rapid ventricular rates, rate control will have to be initiated. Optimally this will encompass the initiation of a beta blocker or a non-dihydropyridine calcium channel blocker. Digoxin is now employed less than in the remote past as it is less effective under most circumstances. Additionally, digitalis can enhance the presence of vagal-induced AF. The use of a beta blocker or alternatively verapamil may provide some rhythm control potential as well in some patients following the termination of AF. In resistant patients, combinations of these agents may be required. In the setting of heart failure the calcium channel blockers are contraindicated as is rapid administration of a beta blocker. Here digitalis may be of value, as is intravenous amiodarone. Typically, intravenous amiodarone will begin to provide rate control following 300–400 mg, whereas a greater dose is required for termination of the AF. If the ventricular rate is not rapid, one will need to know whether it is because of a chronically administered medication or whether it signals intrinsic AV node dysfunction.

2.2.3.2 *Anticoagulation considerations*

The third step in the sequential approach to AF also encompasses decisions regarding anticoagulation. At this stage one must determine if there is an indication for immediate anticoagulation, such as: a patient with an elevated $CHADS_2$ or CHA_2DS_2-VASc score; a patient with AF of greater than 24–48 hours' duration, or uncertain duration; or a patient with embolic symptoms (e.g. stroke or peripheral embolus). In the case of a stroke, determine with the neurologist how soon anticoagulation may be started (i.e. avoidance of risk of 'haemorrhagic transformation').

Cardioversion, whether electrical or pharmacological, with restoration of sinus rhythm is associated with an unacceptable risk of thromboembolism when AF has lasted more than 24–48 hours (the precise relation of embolic risk to AF duration in this range is uncertain). Thus, AF lasting longer than this period of time or AF of uncertain duration requires 3 weeks or more of effective anticoagulation prior to non-emergent cardioversion or necessitates transoesophageal echocardiogram (TOE) guidance if earlier cardioversion is desired. Even with TOE guidance, initiation of anticoagulation with continued administration post conversion is necessary. Elevated thromboembolic risk markers (by $CHADS_2$ or CHA_2DS_2-VASc score) will determine the need for chronic anticoagulation. When urgent cardioversion is needed, as detailed previously in step one, it should not be delayed because of anticoagulation considerations. Conversely, if amiodarone is initiated for rate control, it must be noted that it could produce cardioversion as well, in which case the anticoagulation comments discussed must be adhered to.

2.2.4 **Rhythm control**

The next step in the new AF patient encounter addresses rhythm control. If cardioversion has not been performed urgently, it is appropriate to determine whether it should be considered now. Since paroxysmal AF (PAF) most often terminates within 24 hours, non-urgent intervention for termination can reasonably be deferred for that duration. Thereafter, while PAF may last up to a week before being called persistent AF, early elective cardioversion should be considered if patient symptomatology so dictates. That is, new-onset AF that is tolerated once rate control has been attained may be watched for spontaneous termination or may have non-urgent elective cardioversion scheduled and performed. If, however, AF remains troublesome, early cardioversion with TOE guidance should be employed.

2.2.5 **Non-urgent but early cardioversion**

If cardioversion is determined to be appropriate, its mode will have to be selected: electrical or pharmacological. In part this may depend upon circumstances such as the duration of the AF episode (pharmacological cardioversion efficacy decreases progressively with time and only infrequently works after the first 3–7 days), the patient's fed or fasting state (electrical cardioversion requires intravenous sedation which should not be administered in the fed state), any institution- and country-specific prevailing methods of cardioversion and available pharmaceuticals, and the availability of a physician certified to administer sedation if electric cardioversion is selected.

If pharmacological cardioversion is chosen one must determine whether the patient's status indicates desirability of a more rapid approach (intravenous ibutilide or vernakalant or others—the availability of which is country specific, or whether it can be deferred for several hours such that oral 'pill-in-the-pocket' can be tried (e.g. propafenone, flecainide, ranolazine). If flecainide (300 mg) or propafenone (600 mg immediate-release formulation) are chosen for cardioversion a rate control agent should be given about an hour prior to the AAD (either a beta blocker or a non-dihydropyridine calcium channel blocker, using an immediate-release formulation) so as to protect against rapid rates if atrial flutter were to develop. Digitalis is too slow to use for this purpose in this setting. Ranolazine does not induce atrial flutter and may be given to patients with structural heart disease but experience as 'pill-in-the-pocket' (a 2000 mg dose) is much more limited than that of the class IC agents. However, the class IC agents must be avoided in patients with structural heart disease other than uncomplicated hypertension (no ischaemia, no hypertrophy).

2.2.6 **Antiarrhythmic drug initiation**

Current guidelines suggest that AADs should usually not be started for the first episode of AF. Rather, rate control and anticoagulation as indicated are used. Recurrence patterns as briefly discussed earlier will then determine AAD use. No recurrence = no AAD. Infrequent but tolerated recurrences could be treated with a 'pill-in-the-pocket' antiarrhythmic regimen without chronic AAD administration. Generally the single-dose class IC AAD regimens provided earlier have an average time to conversion of approximately 3–4 hours. Ranolazine appears to average about 6 hours. Recurrences that occur too frequently (as defined by the patient) or are poorly tolerated (such as those with haemodynamic adversity) would be appropriate indications to start a daily AAD regimen.

Before initiating an AAD, whether at the first encounter or a later one, one must determine the patient's profile as regards agents that may be considered and those that should be avoided and also whether there may be a patient-specific profile that could indicate a specific AAD. The American College of Cardiology/American Heart Association/Heart Rhythm Society, the ESC, and other similar organizations have published guidelines with respect to AAD selection for AF. These guidelines favour minimization of organ toxic and proarrhythmic risk over efficacy in deciding the sequence of AADs (or ablation) to be used. I strongly believe that they should be followed unless a specific characteristic in individual patients indicates otherwise. With respect to the latter, the literature supports vagolytic agents (such as disopyramide) for vagal-induced AF, quinidine for AF associated with the Brugada syndrome (with avoidance of other class I AADs), beta blockers as first-line antiarrhythmics in stimulant or catecholamine-induced AF, and perhaps flecainide or ranolazine for AF associated with type 3 long QT syndrome.

Since AADs are generally not initiated with the first-onset AF, these decisions are usually not required during the initial encounter with the new AF patient. However, it may be appropriate to start an AAD if a recurrence is likely and is expected to be poorly tolerated and in specific circumstances where high short-term recurrence rates are likely (e.g. after cardiac surgery, with acute pulmonary disease, with hyperthyroidism). In the latter circumstances the antiarrhythmic can be discontinued when the underlying condition has passed.

When there is an indication for initiating an AAD, one must first also correct any electrolyte disorders that are present. One must also determine if abnormal renal or hepatic function exist, whether there may be interactions with other drugs the patient is taking, and are there ECG patterns that would affect the class of AAD to be considered (sinus node, AV node, intraventricular conduction disorder, prolonged repolarization) as these, too, may affect drug choice, drug dose, and risk.

2.2.7 **Delayed (postponed) cardioversion**

The final step in the initial encounter, step five, is that of deciding to delay (postpone) cardioversion for days or longer. Severe heart failure, acute overwhelming pulmonary disease, thyrotoxicosis, phaeochromocytoma, and the like make achieving and then maintaining sinus rhythm unlikely until they have been treated. In such circumstances if the patient is tolerating the AF upon rate control, cardioversion of the persistent episode should be deferred unless an attempt is necessitated by acute ischaemic or haemodynamic factors and in which case AAD initiation to reduce the likelihood or early recurrence will also need to be utilized. Also at this stage one should complete the evaluation of the patient's underlying conditions if circumstances prevented this earlier or if it requires the scheduling of elective diagnostic tests (Box 2.2).

2.3 **The asymptomatic patient**

In 10–20% of patients with AF, the patient's AF is first detected incidentally. In most circumstances the patient is asymptomatic. In some, the patient has had non-specific symptoms, such as fatigue or dyspnoea, that he/she has ignored or has attributed to some other cause. In still others the AF is detected only upon interrogation of an implanted device (such as a pacemaker or defibrillator). For such patients, aside from decisions regarding chronic anticoagulation (initiate if high-risk thromboembolic markers are present) and rate control (to prevent a tachycardic-induced cardiomyopathy or worsened heart failure, no acute intervention or specific therapy is required at the initial encounter of AF. However patient-specific considerations focus upon whether or not preventive antiarrhythmic therapy is necessary for reasons other than current symptoms and how to judge its efficacy in the absence of AF-associated symptoms.

It is important to note that there we will occasionally encounter a patient for whom pursuit of sinus rhythm is not entertained even if symptomatic. There is a general feeling as well as a consensus expressed in the AFNET/EHRA document that all patients deserve at least one chance of having sinus rhythm restored. However, in rare circumstances when AF is encountered for the first time the decision is made to leave the patient in AF. Such patients might include an incompetent, bed-bound, nursing home patient.

2.3.1 **Site of the first encounter**

Beyond this five-step approach, other patient-specific factors must be addressed at the initial encounter with a new-onset AF patient. They largely relate to the site of the encounter.

If the patient is in the emergency department, a determination must be made as to whether or not to admit the patient to the hospital. Hospitalization may be necessitated by haemodynamic or ischaemic conditions, by concomitant acute precipitating disorders requiring hospitalization for their therapy (such as pulmonary emboli, severe pneumonia, severe pericarditis, etc.), or by the need for continuous ECG monitoring because of the planned initiation of a class III AAD or because the patient has never been seen before and the presence of underlying severe sinus node dysfunction should the AF stop cannot be excluded. However, many patients can be safely discharged to out-patient testing, treatment, and follow-up.

If the patient is in the office one must determine whether or not out-patient management is appropriate. This decision should be based upon how the patient is tolerating the symptoms. The presence of tolerable symptoms and the absence of acute instability may allow rate control and anticoagulation (if warranted) to be initiated as an out-patient with the patient then followed up comfortably with an office visit in 24–48 hours. It is also dependent upon prior information about the patient such that sinus node and conduction system status as well as patient reliability regarding medication compliance and office appointments is known and acceptable.

Lastly, if the patient is first encountered and managed in a setting where a cardiologist is not involved with his or her care, the AFNET/EHRA consensus document clearly indicates that every patient with AF should then be seen by and managed with a cardiologist. This recommendation is based upon repeated evidence that outcomes are better and anticoagulation use is more frequently and appropriately employed by and continued by cardiologists than by primary care physicians.

2.4 Conclusion to what should be done when atrial fibrillation first presents

AF is growing dramatically in prevalence and will continue to do so progressively. For every patient with AF, there is a first episode (new onset); and, for most of these the presentation is symptomatic. For all patients with AF considerations, include at a minimum: is there an identifiable/reversible cause; are there underlying contributing co-morbid conditions requiring concomitant therapy; how best to control the ventricular rate; is the patient at low enough risk not to require anticoagulation (most are at risk and do require anticoagulation); which anticoagulant to use; is rhythm therapy required and if so, which approaches and options should be considered. Not all of these are issues that can be addressed at the first visit; however, some can and all must be considered. In addition, unique to new-onset AF, are additional considerations regarding hospitalization versus out-patient management and who will be the primary managing care-giver. The chapter addresses in detail these issues as they apply to the new-onset AF patient and, hopefully, will provide the reader a measure of clinical confidence regarding the initial evaluation required and the initial management choices to be made.

Key reading

Abusaada K, Sharma SB, Jaladi R, Ezekowitz MD. Epidemiology and management of new-onset atrial fibrillation. *Am J Managed Care* 2004; 10(3 Suppl): S50–7.

Buccelletti F, Di Somma S, Galante A, Pugliese F, Alegiani F, Bertazzoni G, *et al*. Disparities in management of new-onset atrial fibrillation in the emergency department despite adherence to the current guidelines: data from a large metropolitan area. *Intern Emerg Med* 2011; 6(2): 149–56.

Dell'Orfano JT, Patel H, Wolbrette DL, Luck JC, Naccarelli GV. Acute treatment of atrial fibrillation: spontaneous conversion rates and cost of care. *Am J Cardiol* 1999; 83: 788–90.

European Heart Rhythm Association, European Association for Cardio-Thoracic Surgery, Camm AJ, Kirchhof P, Lip GY, Schotten U, *et al*. Guidelines for the management of atrial fibrillation: the Task Force for the Management of Atrial Fibrillation of the European Society of Cardiology (ESC). *Eur Heart J* 2010; 31(19): 2369–429.

Fuster V, Ryden LE, Asinger RW, Cannom DS, Crijns HJ, Frye RL, et al. ACC/AHA/ESC guidelines for the management of patients with atrial fibrillation. A report of the American College of Cardiology/American Heart Association Task Force on Practice Guidelines and the European Society of Cardiology Committee for Practice Guidelines and Policy Conferences (Committee to develop guidelines for the management of patients with atrial fibrillation) developed in collaboration with the North American Society of Pacing and Electrophysiology. Eur Heart J 2001; 22(20): 1852–923.

Fuster V, Ryden LE, Cannom DS, Criijns HJ, Curtis AB, Ellenbogen KA, et al. 2011 ACCF/AHA/HRS focused updates incorporated into the ACC/AHA/ESC 2006 Guidelines for the management of patients with atrial fibrillation: a report of the American College of Cardiology Foundation/American Heart Association Task Force on Practice Guidelines developed in partnership with the European Society of Cardiology and in collaboration with the European Heart Rhythm Association and the Heart Rhythm Society. J Am Coll Cardiol 2011; 57(11): e101–98.

Fuster V, Ryden LE, Cannom DS, Crijns HJ, Curtis AB, Ellenbogen KA, et al. 2011 ACCF/AHA/HRS focused updates incorporated into the ACC/AHA/ESC 2006 guidelines for the management of patients with atrial fibrillation: a report of the American College of Cardiology Foundation/American Heart Association Task Force on practice guidelines. Circulation 2011; 123(10): e269–367.

Fuster V, Ryden LE, Cannom DS, Crijns HJ, Curtis AB, Ellenbogen KA, et al. ACC/AHA/ESC 2006 guidelines for the management of patients with atrial fibrillation: full text: a report of the American College of Cardiology/American Heart Association Task Force on practice guidelines and the European Society of Cardiology Committee for Practice Guidelines (Writing Committee to Revise the 2001 guidelines for the management of patients with atrial fibrillation) developed in collaboration with the European Heart Rhythm Association and the Heart Rhythm Society. Europace 2006; 8(9): 651–745.

Gillis AM, Skanes AC. Comparing the 2010 North American and European atrial fibrillation guidelines Can J Cardiol 2011; 27(1): 7–13.

Katsnelson M, Sacco RL, Moscucci M. Progress for stroke prevention with atrial fibrillation: emergence of alternative oral anticoagulants. Stroke 2012; 43(4): 1179–85.

Kirchhof P, Breithardt G, Aliot E, Al Khatib S, Apostolakis S, Auricchio A, et al. Personalized management of atrial fibrillation: Proceedings from the fourth Atrial Fibrillation competence NETwork/European Heart Rhythm Association consensus conference Europace 2013; doi: 10.1093/europace/eut232

Lackland DT, Elkind MS, D'Agostino R Sr, Dhamoon MS, Goff DC Jr, Higashida RT, et al. Inclusion of stroke in cardiovascular risk prediction instruments: a statement for healthcare professionals from the American Heart Association/American Stroke Association. Stroke 2012; 43(7): 1998–2027.

LaHaye SA, Gibbens SL, Ball DG, Day AG, Olesen JB, Skanes AC. A clinical decision aid for the selection of antithrombotic therapy for the prevention of stroke due to atrial fibrillation. Eur Heart J 2012 33(17): 2163–71.

LeLorier P, Klein GJ, Krahn A, Yee R, Skanes A. Should patients with asymptomatic Wolff–Parkinson–White pattern undergo a catheter ablation? Curr Cardiol Rep 2001; 3(4): 301–4.

Lip GY, Andreotti F, Fauchier L, Huber K, Hylek E, Knight E, et al. Bleeding risk assessment and management in atrial fibrillation patients. Executive Summary of a Position Document from the European Heart Rhythm Association [EHRA], endorsed by the European Society of Cardiology [ESC] Working Group on Thrombosis. Thromb Haemost 2011; 106(6): 997–1011.

Marinelli A, Capucci A. Antiarrhythmic drugs for atrial fibrillation. Expert Opin Pharmacother 2011 12(8): 1201–15.

Murdock DK, Reiffel JA, Kaliebe J, Larrain G. Electrophysiological changes of the atrium in patients with lone paroxysmal atrial fibrillation. JAFIB 2010; 3(2): 10–13.

Reiffel JA. Selecting an antiarrhythmic agent for atrial fibrillation should be a patient-specific, data-driven decision. Am J Cardiol 1998; 82(8A): 72N–81N.

Reiffel JA. Have sanctioned algorithms replaced empiric judgment in the selection process of antiarrhythmic drugs for the therapy for atrial fibrillation? Curr Cardiol Rep 2004; 6(5): 365–70.

Reiffel JA. A contemporary look at classic trials in atrial fibrillation: what do they really show and how might they apply to future therapies? Am J Cardiol 2008; 102(6A): 3H–11H.

Reiffel JA. Cardioversion for atrial fibrillation: treatment options and advances. PACE 2009 32(8): 1073–84.

Reiffel JA. Atrial fibrillation: what have recent trials taught us regarding pharmacologic management of rate and rhythm control? PACE 2011; 34(2): 247–59.

Reiffel JA, Naccarelli GV. Antiarrhythmic drug therapy for atrial fibrillation: are the guidelines guiding clinical practice? *Clin Cardiol* 2006; 29(3): 97–102.

Savelieva I, Camm AJ. Clinical relevance of silent atrial fibrillation: prevalence, prognosis, quality of life, and management. *J Intervent Cardiac Electrophysiol* 2000; 4(2): 369–82.

Skanes AC, Healey JS, Cairns JA, Dorian P, Gillis AM, McMurtry MS, *et al.* Focused 2012 update of the Canadian Cardiovascular Society atrial fibrillation guidelines: recommendations for stroke prevention and rate/rhythm control. *Can J Cardiol* 2012; 28(2): 125–36.

You JJ, Singer DE, Howard PA, Lane DA, Eckman MH, Fang MC, *et al.* Antithrombotic therapy for atrial fibrillation: Antithrombotic Therapy and Prevention of Thrombosis, 9th ed: American College of Chest Physicians Evidence-Based Clinical Practice Guidelines. *Chest* 2012; 141(Suppl 2): e531S–575S.

Chapter 3

Workup for patients with atrial fibrillation

Bart A. Mulder and Isabelle C. Van Gelder

Key points

- Screening for atrial fibrillation (AF) in the elderly is important to reduce the risk for stroke.
- Anamnesis is key in diagnosing type and severity of the associated symptoms of AF and guides AF therapy.
- Adequate search for underlying (heart) disease is essential for optimal treatment. Prognosis depends on it.
- Left atrial volume is indicative for success of a rhythm control strategy and also for prognosis.
- Assessment of CHA_2DS_2-VASc and HAS-BLED scores for stroke and bleeding risk is indicated in every patient and guides anticoagulation therapy.

3.1 Introduction to workup for patients with atrial fibrillation

Atrial fibrillation (AF) is the most common cardiac arrhythmia and is associated with increased risk of stroke, heart failure, hospitalizations, and death. It is estimated that AF will affect up to 3% of the population by the year 2050. After the age of 40 years one out of four people will develop AF during their remaining lifetime. To manage this upcoming healthcare burden it is important to focus on screening of AF (as 30% is asymptomatic), identifying underlying (heart) disease and precipitating factors, optimally treat the underlying disease, and finally perform risk stratification for stroke and other thromboembolic complications before starting treatment of AF itself.

3.2 How to investigate patients with suspected AF

AF is the main contributor for stroke in the elderly. Therefore, it is important to actively screen patients for AF. Recent studies with implanted devices have shown that AF often occurs asymptomatically, especially in the elderly. Only 6 minutes of AF increased the risk for stroke by 2.5 in a study performed in patients with an increased risk for stroke and an indication for an implantable cardioverter defibrillator or pacemaker. This implies that screening for AF and starting anticoagulation is of major importance for the prognosis (Table 3.1).

Recent AF guidelines suggest that by means of pulse palpitation any nurse or physician should perform opportunistic screening for AF. If AF is suggested or if the patient has complaints of palpitations or other AF-associated symptoms (i.e. dyspnoea) a 12-lead

Table 3.1 Recommendations for diagnosis and initial management

	Recommendation and Level of Evidence
The diagnosis of AF requires documentation by ECG.	1B
In patients with suspected AF, an attempt to record an ECG should be made when symptoms suggestive of AF occur.	1B
A simple symptom score (EHRA score) is recommended to quantify AF-related symptoms.	1B
All patients with AF should undergo a thorough physical examination, and a cardiac- and arrhythmia-related history should be taken.	1C
In patients with severe symptoms, documented or suspected heart disease, or risk factors, an ECG is recommended.	1B
In patients treated with antiarrhythmic drugs, a 12-lead ECG should be recorded at regular intervals during follow-up.	1C

AF = atrial fibrillation; ECG = electrocardiogram; EHRA = European Heart Rhythm Association.

Class 1 = evidence and/or general agreement that a given treatment or procedure is beneficial, useful, effective. B = data derived from a single randomized clinical trial or large non-randomized studies. C = consensus of opinion of the experts and/or small studies, retrospective studies, registries.

Source data from Camm AJ, Kirchhof P, Lip GY, Schotten U, Savelieva I, Ernst S, *et al.* Guidelines for the management of atrial fibrillation: the Task Force for the Management of Atrial Fibrillation of the European Society of Cardiology (ESC). *Europace* 2010; 12: 1360–420.

electrocardiogram is needed to verify the diagnosis (Table 3.1). If a patient has an anamnesis suggesting episodes of paroxysmal AF then the next step may be to perform a 24-hour Holter monitoring or telemonitoring to confirm paroxysmal episodes of AF.

3.2.1 Medical history

AF symptoms include palpitations, dyspnoea, chest pain, and dizziness. Less common complaints are presyncope and syncope. Also symptoms may change over time in the individual patient. During anamnesis several questions are important: is the rhythm irregular or regular, sudden start, are the episodes frequent or infrequent, duration of episodes, does it spontaneously stop, does it start during rest or exercise or during the night, and what are their precipitating factors (e.g. coffee, alcohol, endurance training, sleep, rest, post-prandial)? (Box 3.1). AF may be self-limiting (paroxysmal), or persistent (lasting > 7 days, or needing chemical or electrical cardioversion), or permanent when cardioversion has failed or restoration of sinus rhythm is no longer necessary. Anamnesis combined with the medical history often has clues whether or not a patient has underlying (heart) disease. Has the patient a medical history of heart failure, angina, previous myocardial infarction, chronic obstructive pulmonary disease, valve disease, hyperthyroidism, or peripheral vascular disease? The anamnesis should also include asking for symptoms of underlying heart diseases and triggers. It is important to identify any underlying disease or precipitating factors as these are the basis of AF management. Evaluation should also include determination the European Heart Rhythm Association score for AF-associated symptoms (Table 3.2). This is a straightforward symptom score allowing the physician to gain insight to what extent AF limits a patient in his everyday life and helps to decide whether a rate or rhythm control therapy is indicated. In elderly patients AF can present with symptoms of dizziness and (pre)syncope, and palpitation, when AF occurs in the setting of a bradycardia-tachycardia syndrome.

Box 3.1 Relevant questions to be put to a patient with suspected or known AF
• Does the heart rhythm during the episode feel regular or irregular? • Is there any precipitating factor such as exercise, emotion, or alcohol? • Are symptoms during the episodes moderate or severe?—the severity may be expressed using the European Heart Rhythm Association score (Table 3.2). • Are the episodes frequent or infrequent, and are they long- or short-lasting? • Is there a history of concomitant disease such as hypertension, coronary heart disease, heart failure, peripheral vascular disease, cerebrovascular disease, stroke, diabetes, or chronic pulmonary disease? • Is there an alcohol abuse habit? • Is there a family history of AF?
Reprinted with permission from Camm AJ, Kirchhof P, Lip GY, Schotten U, Savelieva I, Ernst S, *et al.* Guidelines for the management of atrial fibrillation: the Task Force for the Management of Atrial Fibrillation of the European Society of Cardiology (ESC). *Europace* 2010; 12: 1360–420 by permission of Oxford University Press.

3.2.2 **Physical examination and laboratory analyses**

After the anamnesis it is essential to perform a thorough physical examination including length, weight and body mass index, blood pressure, heart rate (regular or irregular), palpitation of the thyroid gland and other signs of hyperthyroidism (skin, nails, and hair), assessment of the jugular venous pulse, auscultation of the heart and lungs for murmurs and underlying lung disease or rales, and inspection of legs, ankles, and abdomen for oedema and signs of vascular disease.

At that moment additional laboratory testing is of help: thyroid stimulating hormone, haemoglobin, fasting glucose (or HbA1c), sodium, potassium, serum creatinine, liver function tests, cholesterol levels, and if available N-terminal prohormone of brain natriuretic peptide (NT-proBNP) to find evidence for underlying (heart) disease and prognosis.

3.2.3 **Twelve-lead electrocardiogram**

The 12-lead electrocardiogram does not only provide information about the heart rhythm. It may also help to find underlying (heart) diseases. First, if a patient has sinus rhythm on the electrocardiogram assessment of p-wave morphology can give clues for enlarged atria which can be verified by echocardiography. This is clinically relevant because patients with enlarged atria show lower long-term success of rhythm control therapy. Secondly,

Table 3.2 Classification of AF-related symptoms: European Heart Rhythm Association (EHRA) score	
EHRA I	No symptoms
EHRA II	Mild symptoms; normal daily activity not affected
EHRA III	Severe symptoms; normal daily activity affected
EHRA IV	Disabling symptoms; normal daily activity discontinued
Reprinted with permission from Camm AJ, Kirchhof P, Lip GY, Schotten U, Savelieva I, Ernst S, *et al.* Guidelines for the management of atrial fibrillation: the Task Force for the Management of Atrial Fibrillation of the European Society of Cardiology (ESC). *Europace* 2010; 12: 1360–420 by permission of Oxford University Press.	

intraventricular conduction disturbances can be assessed which can be seen as a wide QRS (≥120 milliseconds) complex on the electrocardiogram. This may be a sign of structural heart disease. Q waves may be a sign of prior myocardial infarction. A delta wave or short PR interval are signs of pre-excitation and assessment of voltage criteria for left ventricular hypertrophy are relevant because they may also point to underlying heart diseases.

3.3 Who needs additional testing?

Most of the patients with new-onset AF should be consulted by a cardiologist at least once (Table 3.1). It is important to examine for underlying (heart) disease and start adequate therapy accordingly. Only in elderly patients does it seem justified to start treatment for AF by the general practitioner.

3.3.1 Transthoracic echocardiogram and cardiac stress test

An echocardiogram is important in the workup of patients with AF. In fact, every patient with new-onset AF should undergo a transthoracic echocardiogram to identify underlying heart diseases. It is helpful since it provides essential information about the anatomy and functioning of the heart. It identifies atrial, ventricular, and valvular diseases as well as previous unidentified congenital heart diseases. An important assessment in patients with AF is the left atrial volume since it reflects the stretch of the left atrium and thus is an important marker of underlying disease (i.e. hypertension, mitral valve disease, left ventricular dysfunction). An enlarged left atrial volume has important prognostic significance. It is not only an important predictor of cardiovascular events but also for maintenance of sinus rhythm. If the left atrium is enlarged the patient will be more likely to have recurrences of AF. Assessment of left ventricular function is also useful as some antiarrhythmic and rate control drugs are contraindicated in patients with a reduced ejection fraction (e.g. non-dihydropyridine calcium channel blockers like verapamil). A transoesophageal echocardiogram is seldom indicated. A cardiac stress test is useful in patients presenting with signs or risk factors for coronary artery disease. It also provides essential information about heart rate and blood pressure during exercise.

3.4 The search for underlying heart disease

3.4.1 Hypertension

The prognosis of AF is mainly dependent on the underlying heart disease. Therefore it is important to look for risk factors for AF. Hypertension is one of the most important risk factors not only as far as AF itself is concerned but also for AF-related complications, especially stroke and heart failure. Hypertension is probably one of the most underestimated diseases of our time and treatment is often not instituted at an early stage.

3.4.2 Valvular disease

Valvular disease is also a well-known risk factor for AF. While rheumatic valve disease is not common any more in the Western world there are parts of the world where it still is frequently encountered. All valvular lesions with significant regurgitation or stenosis can lead to AF. Mitral stenosis and mitral regurgitation can lead to dilatation of the left atrium and thereby increasing risk for AF. Aortic valve disease may cause atrial remodelling due to increasing atrial stretch and thereby increasing atrial volume secondary to left ventricular overload.

3.4.3 Heart failure

There is a mutual relation between heart failure and AF. This can be explained by the presence of shared risk factors such as age, hypertension, as well as valvular disease and an old myocardial infarction. Heart failure may set the stage for AF because of changes in the atrial myocardium, that is, structural remodelling in combination with electrophysiological changes. Due to uncontrolled high heart rates, an irregular ventricular rhythm, loss of atrioventricular synchrony, an increase of atrioventricular regurgitation, and the absence of filling of the left ventricle due to loss of atrial kick, AF may induce heart failure or further deteriorate heart failure.

Survival of acute myocardial infarction has dramatically increased since the introduction of percutaneous coronary intervention. As a consequence fewer patients will develop heart failure with reduced ejection fraction below 35–40%. Nowadays heart failure with preserved ejection fraction due to advancing age and hypertension contributes to almost 50% of all new cases of chronic heart failure and AF is common in these patients (~30%).

3.4.4 Coronary artery disease

In patients with stable coronary artery disease AF is commonly encountered. In the setting of an old myocardial infarction the occurrence of AF is associated with an impaired left ventricle systolic and diastolic function. Another trigger may be ischaemia. Therefore, exclusion of significant coronary artery disease is essential in patients presenting with AF.

3.5 Important risk factors beyond the heart

3.5.1 Thyroid disease

Overt hyperthyroidism is an important cause of AF, and may increase the risk of incident AF. Several large community-based studies showed that the incidence of AF within populations with overt hyperthyroidism increased with age, and with a peak-incidence in individuals older than 70 years. Around 10–25% of patients with hyperthyroidism have AF and it is most commonly observed in men and the elderly. Laboratory testing for hyperthyroidism is important as successful treatment of hyperthyroidism to a euthyroid state often results in reversion to sinus rhythm (55–75%). Also subclinical hyperthyroidism (normal thyrotropin with elevated thyroxine and/or triiodothyronine) is an important risk factor and may increase AF risk in an extent similar to overt hyperthyroidism.

3.5.2 Obesity

Several observations in community- and hospital-based studies have related obesity (defined as body mass index > 30 kg/m^2), with AF. Obesity may increase the risk for AF by several mechanisms. First, obesity has been associated with diastolic dysfunction, elevated plasma volume, and increased neurohormonal activation resulting in stretch and dilatation of the left atrium. Secondly, obesity may predispose to obstructive sleep apnoea syndrome and autonomic dysfunction, both also associated with AF. Finally, adipose tissue itself has been related to the development of cardiovascular diseases and AF, through secretion of pro-inflammatory cytokines and adipokines. Therefore patients need to be educated that weight loss may result in prevention of AF.

3.5.3 Obstructive sleep apnoea

Obstructive sleep apnoea (OSA) can be found in at least 10–15% of patients presenting with AF. AF and OSA share similar characteristics and underlying diseases: hypertension, male sex, older age, and increased body mass index. Detection and adequate therapy of OSA may reduce AF burden.

3.5.4 Diabetes mellitus

Diabetes is frequently encountered in patients with AF. The exact mechanisms by which diabetes increases the risk for AF remain unknown. However, it is probably related to the cardiovascular complications associated with diabetes. In patients with diabetes AF is associated with adverse prognosis with an increase in cardiovascular events and death. Diabetes is also important as it is a major contributing factor for stroke and anticoagulation therapy might therefore be of recommended.

3.6 CHA_2DS_2-VASc and HAS-BLED risk scores

The search for underlying heart disease is not only of importance for the treatment of AF but also to assess the risk for stroke and bleeding. AF manifests not only as an electrical disease but also as a hypercoagulable disease. The relationship between AF and vascular risks centres on activation of blood coagulation. Strokes in AF patients frequently originate from the left atrium which becomes particularly thrombogenic after AF has developed. Nonetheless emboli can also originate from arterial vessels. To overcome this deleterious complication several stroke risk schemes have been introduced in the last few years of which currently the CHA_2DS_2-VASc score is used to identify those patients benefiting the most from anticoagulation treatment (Table 3.3). When a patient has two or more risk factors oral anticoagulation should be initiated. In case of a CHA_2DS_2-VASc score of 0 the preferred choice is to start no anticoagulation. In patients with a CHA_2DS_2-VASc score of 1 either no anticoagulation or oral anticoagulation can be initiated. Another risk assessment in the workup is to assess bleeding risk (Table 3.4). This can be done with the HAS-BLED risk scheme of which several risk factors are similar to the CHA_2DS_2-VASc score but there are some differences: abnormal kidney or liver function, previous bleeding, and labile INRs. When a patient had a HAS-BLED score of 3 or higher there is a high risk for bleeding. This does not imply that there is a contraindication for anticoagulation, merely that regular follow-ups are necessary and institution with anticoagulation should be performed with caution. It is important to realize that stroke risk is often underestimated while bleeding

Table 3.3 CHA_2DS_2-VASc score	
Risk factor	Score
Congestive heart failure/left ventricular dysfunction	1
Hypertension	1
Age ≥ 75 years	2
Diabetes mellitus	1
Stroke/transient ischaemic attack/thromboembolism	2
Vascular disease	1
Age 65–74	1
Sex **c**ategory	1

Source data from Camm AJ, Kirchhof P, Lip GY, Schotten U, Savelieva I, Ernst S, et al. Guidelines for the management of atrial fibrillation: the Task Force for the Management of Atrial Fibrillation of the European Society of Cardiology (ESC). *Europace* 2010; 12: 1360–420.

Table 3.4 HAS-BLED score

Risk factor	Score	Definition
Hypertension	1	Systolic blood pressure ≥ 160 mmHg
Abnormal renal and liver function (1 point each)	1 or 2	Chronic dialysis; renal transplantation; serum creatinine ≥ 200 mmol/L Chronic hepatic disease; bilirubin 2× or 3× normal with ALT, AST, or alkaline phosphatase 3× normal
Stroke	1	History of stroke
Bleeding	1	History of bleeding or predisposition to bleeding
Labile INRs	1	Unstable/high INRs or time in therapeutic range < 60%
Elderly	1	Age > 65 years
Drugs or alcohol (1 point each)	1 or 2	Concomitant use of aspirin or NSAID, ≥ 8 units/week

ALT = alanine aminotransferase; AST = aspartate aminotransferase; INR = international normalized ratio; NSAID = non-steroidal anti-inflammatory drug.

Source data from Pisters R, Lane DA, Nieuwlaat R, de Vos CB, Crijns HJ, Lip GY. A novel user friendly score (HAS-BLED) to assess one-year risk of major bleeding in atrial fibrillation patients: The Euro Heart Survey. *Chest* 2010; 138: 1093–100.

risk is often overestimated. It is noteworthy that the intracranial haemorrhage (and major bleeding) rate in patients on aspirin, for a given HAS-BLED score, was similar to that for those taking warfarin. Nevertheless the physician should be careful and these risk scores can provide a handle to work with.

3.7 Clinical pearls

- Educate your patients and your staff.
- AF is not a benign disease and is associated with increased morbidity and mortality.
- Treat hypertension early as it is the most important risk factor for AF and stroke.
- Re-assess CHA_2DS_2VASc and HAS-BLED scores yearly for up-to-date stroke and bleeding risk.

Key reading

Camm AJ, Kirchhof P, Lip GY, Schotten U, Savelieva I, Ernst S, *et al*. Guidelines for the management of atrial fibrillation: the Task Force for the Management of Atrial Fibrillation of the European Society of Cardiology (ESC). *Europace* 2010; 12: 1360–420.

Camm AJ, Lip GY, De Caterina R, Savelieva I, Atar D, Hohnloser SH, *et al*. 2012 focused update of the ESC Guidelines for the management of atrial fibrillation: an update of the 2010 ESC Guidelines for the management of atrial fibrillation. Developed with the special contribution of the European Heart Rhythm Association. *Europace* 2012; 14: 1385–413.

Dahlöf B, Devereux RB, Kjeldsen SE, Julius S, Beevers G, de Faire U, *et al*; LIFEStudy Group. Cardiovascular morbidity and mortality in the Losartan Intervention For Endpoint reduction in hypertension study (LIFE): a randomised trial against atenolol. *Lancet* 2002; 359: 995–1003.

Dorian P, Jung W, Newman D, Paquette M, Wood K, Ayers GM, *et al*. The impairment of health-related quality of life in patients with intermittent atrial fibrillation: implications for the assessment of investigational therapy. *J Am Coll Cardiol* 2000; 36: 1303–9.

Gerdts E, Wachtell K, Omvik P, Otterstad JE, Oikarinen L, Boman K, *et al*. Left atrial size and risk of major cardiovascular events during antihypertensive treatment: losartan intervention for endpoint reduction in hypertension trial. *Hypertension* 2007; 49: 311–16.

Healey JS, Connolly SJ, Gold MR, Israel CW, Van Gelder IC, Capucci A, *et al*, ASSERT Investigators. Subclinical atrial fibrillation and the risk of stroke. *N Engl J Med* 2012; 366: 120–9.

Heidbuchel H, Verhamme P, Alings M, Antz M, Hacke W, Oldgren J, *et al*. European Heart Rhythm Association Practical Guide on the use of new oral anticoagulants in patients with non-valvular atrial fibrillation. *Europace* 2013; 15(5): 625–51.

Hijazi Z, Oldgren J, Andersson U, Connolly SJ, Ezekowitz MD, Hohnloser SH, *et al*. Cardiac biomark-ers are associated with an increased risk of stroke and death in patients with atrial fibrillation: a Randomized Evaluation of Long-term Anticoagulation Therapy (RE-LY) substudy. *Circulation* 2012; 125: 1605–16.

Lau CP, Gbadebo TD, Connolly SJ, Van Gelder IC, Capucci A, Gold MR, *et al.*; ASSERT investiga-tors. Ethnic differences in atrial fibrillation identified using implanted cardiac devices. *J Cardiovasc Electrophysiol* 2013; 24: 381–7

Lip GY, Nieuwlaat R, Pisters R, Lane DA, Crijns HJ. Refining clinical risk stratification for predicting stroke and thromboembolism in atrial fibrillation using a novel risk factor-based approach: the Euro Heart Survey on atrial fibrillation. *Chest* 2010; 137: 263–72.

Mancia G, Fagard R, Narkiewicz K, Redon J, Zanchetti A, Böhm M, *et al*. 2013 ESH/ESC Guidelines for the management of arterial hypertension: The Task Force for the management of arterial hyperten-sion of the European Society of Hypertension and of the European Society of Cardiology. *Eur Heart J* 2013; 34(28): 2159–219.

Neuberger HR, Mewis C, van Veldhuisen DJ, Schotten U, van Gelder IC, Allessie MA, *et al*. Management of atrial fibrillation in patients with heart failure. *Eur Heart J* 2007; 28: 2568–77.

Pisters R, Lane DA, Nieuwlaat R, de Vos CB, Crijns HJ, Lip GY. A novel user friendly score (HAS-BLED) to assess one-year risk of major bleeding in atrial fibrillation patients: The Euro Heart Survey. *Chest* 2010; 138: 1093–100.

Rienstra M, Van Gelder IC, Hagens VE, Veeger NJ, Van Veldhuisen DJ, Crijns HJ. Mending the rhythm does not improve prognosis in patients with persistent atrial fibrillation: a subanalysis of the RACE study. *Eur Heart J* 2006; 27: 357–64.

Schoonderwoerd BA, Smit MD, Pen L, Van Gelder IC. New risk factors for atrial fibrillation: Causes of 'not-so-lone atrial fibrillation'. *Europace* 2008; 10: 668–73.

Smit MD, Moes ML, Maass AH, Achekar ID, Van Geel PP, Hillege HL, *et al*. The importance of whether atrial fibrillation or heart failure develops first. *Eur J Heart Fail* 2012; 14: 1030–40.

Smit MD, Van Gelder IC. New treatment options for atrial fibrillation: towards patient tailored therapy. *Heart* 2011; 97: 1796–802

Van Gelder IC, Hagens VE, Bosker HA, Kingma JH, Kamp O, Kingma T, *et al*. A comparison of rate control and rhythm control in patients with recurrent persistent atrial fibrillation. *N Engl J Med* 2002; 347: 1834–40.

Wyse DG, Waldo AL, DiMarco JP, Domanski MJ, Rosenberg Y, Schron EB, *et al*. A comparison of rate control and rhythm control in patients with atrial fibrillation. *N Engl J Med* 2002; 347: 1825–33.

Chapter 4

Atrial fibrillation in
different clinical subsets

Mohammad Shenasa, Hossein Shenasa,
and Shahrzad Rouhani

Key points

- Atrial fibrillation (AF) is the most common sustained arrhythmia with
  significant morbidity and mortality.

- AF is an age-dependent complex disease with diverse and often concomitant
  aetiologies.

- Although mitral stenosis, alcohol, and thyrotoxicosis are the classic causes of
  AF, hypertension is the most common cause followed by heart failure (HF)
  and coronary artery disease. These aetiologies often coexist.

- HF and stroke are the most devastating complications of AF.

- Emerging risk factors such as endurance athletics, obesity, obstructive sleep
  apnoea, and impaired renal function complicate management of AF.

- Asymptomatic 'silent' AF poses as significant a risk of adverse effects as
  symptomatic AF, for example, stroke.

- AF is an independent risk factor for sudden cardiac death.

- In young patients (< 60 years old) with AF without any detectable structural
  heart diseases (lone AF), screening of family members for genetically related
  AF and other inherited arrhythmias is recommended.

- Management should target detection and modification of underlying causes
  and co-morbidities, and prevent or delay recurrence and progression of AF
  and its complications.

4.1 Introduction to atrial fibrillation in different
clinical subsets

Atrial fibrillation (AF) is the most common sustained rhythm disorder encountered in clinical
practice and is a heterogeneous disease with many aetiologies, as shown in Figure 4.1. Table
4.1 summarizes the risk factors and markers for AF. The arrhythmia is associated with high
morbidity and mortality rates and has a significant social and economic burden. Its mechanisms, natural history, prognosis, management, response to therapy, and outcomes are
highly variable and for most patients depend upon the underlying heart disease(s) and the
rate of progression. More than 80% of patients with AF have one or multiple structural heart
diseases (SHD). Many of these pathologies produce atrial remodelling, inflammation, and

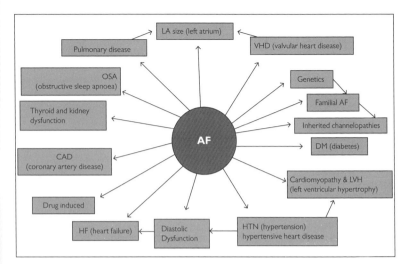

Figure 4.1 Common aetiologies of atrial fibrillation (AF). Modified with permission from Mohammad Shenasa, Mona Soleimanieh, Fatemah Shenasa, Individualized therapy in patients with atrial fibrillation: new look at atrial fibrillation, *Europace* 2012; 14: v121–4 by permission of Oxford University Press.

fibrosis, which are the final common pathways for the genesis and maintenance of AF. The lifetime risk of developing AF for both men and women after the age of 40 years is one in four (26% for men and 23% for women), which is high compared to other cardiovascular and non-cardiovascular diseases. AF is an age-dependent disease and after the age of 60, the risk of AF double with each decade of life. Age by itself produces atrial fibrosis, extensive senile amyloid infiltration, left atrial enlargement, diastolic dysfunction, and reduced left atrial appendage flow velocity, all of which are predisposing factors for AF. AF is more prevalent in males than in females; however, new-onset AF increases the risk of death and cardiovascular events such as stroke in women more than in men (Conen et al. 2011; Perez et al. 2013). Currently, it is estimated that 1.5–2% of the general population suffers from AF and there are 2.3 million patients in the United States and 6 million in Europe with AF. It is projected that by 2030 there will be 12.1 million in the United States and by 2050 the numbers will be between 5.6 million to as high as 15.9 million (Go et al. 2001, 2003, Olesen et al. 2011 and Roger et al. 2012). A more recent report projected that the number of patients with AF in the European Union from 2010 to 2060 in adults over 55 years of age will be 17.9 million (Krijthe et al. 2013 and Chin and Win-Kuang 2007). AF currently accounts for one-third of hospitalization due to cardiac arrhythmias; however, the magnitude of these projections may be underestimated due to many episodes of asymptomatic AF. Kim et al. (2011) recently reported in a Medicare population, that the estimated total incremental annual healthcare cost in patients with AF is $6–26.0 billion (about $8705 per patient in 2008).

Although we have witnessed more than a century of experience with AF, and have had many breakthroughs, our strategies in prevention and treatment have remained unsatisfactory (Fye 2006 and Prystowsky 2008). This in part may be related to the complexity of AF by itself and/or its interrelationship with many other SHDs and genetic and environmental factors, as well as systemic co-morbidities. The limitations so far could also be due to the fact that arrhythmia management has been focused on mechanisms based on experimental models rather than aetiology. The recent paradigm shift towards aetiology and

Table 4.1 Risk factors, clinical conditions, and biomarkers for the development of AF

Traditional risk factors	Novel risk factors	Biomarkers
Age, male sex	Reduced vascular compliance	Increased arterial stiffness
Hypertension/diabetes mellitus	Atherosclerosis	Prolonged QRS duration
Alcohol consumption/smoking	Insulin resistance	P-wave dispersion
Clinical conditions	Environmental factors (air pollution etc.)	Low birthweight
LVH	Excess vitamin D	Inflammatory markers
Myocardial infarction/HF	atrial fibrosis	Neurohormones
Valvular heart disease	Antiarrhythmic agents	Genetic variants
Thyroid disease	Extreme exercise	Pulse pressure
Prior cardiac surgery/post-cardiac surgery	Inflammation oxidative stress	Thyroid stimulation hormone, T3, T4
Congenital heart disease	Obstructive sleep apnoea	ANP
Cardiomyopathies	Obesity/metabolic syndrome	Hs-CRP
Inherited channelopathies	Air pollution (Link et al. 2013)	Interleukin-6
Autonomic imbalance	Gout	Angiotensin II
Chronic kidney disease		Markers for fibrosis
Electrolyte imbalance		mRNA (De Souza and Camm 2012)
Pulmonary disease		
Echocardiographic predictors of AF		
		LV fractional shortening
		Mitral annular calcification
		Left atrial enlargement
		LVH (LV wall thickness)

ANP = atrial natriuretic peptide; HF = heart failure; Hs-CRP = high sensitivity C-reactive protein; LV = left ventricle; LVH = left ventricular hypertrophy.

evidence-based personalized AF management should lower its global burden. There are also concerns regarding guideline implementation and treatment adherence. A recent report by Hess et al. (2013) on the use of evidence-based cardiac prevention therapy among outpatients with AF demonstrated that the majority of eligible AF outpatients did not receive all guideline-recommended therapies for cardiovascular comorbid conditions and risk factors.

The pathophysiological and cellular mechanisms of AF depend on triggers that often originate in the pulmonary veins or within the atria, its interaction with substrates located in the left and/or right atrium, the presence of either focal or multiple re-entrant wavelets or a single driver, and neurohormonal modulators. This discussion is beyond the scope and purpose of this review and is well discussed in the articles by Wakili et al. (2011), Iwasaki et al. (2011), and Nattel and Harada (2014).

4.1.1 **Definitions of AF**

AF is a supraventricular tachyarrhythmia (SVT) diagnosed from an electrocardiogram (ECG) and is characterized by an absence of a well-defined P wave and an irregularly irregular RR interval without a recurring pattern. Fibrillatory waves often are noted that vary in amplitude, shape, and timing, and may be more dominant (> 1 mm referred to as coarse AF, and < 1 mm referred to as fine AF). The atrial rate in AF is very rapid, usually more than 300 beats per minute (varies between 300 and 600), disorganized, and mechanically ineffective. Figures 4.2, 4.3 and 4.4 demonstrate the different ECG types of AF and associated arrythmias.

AF burden is a measure of the proportion of time spent in AF. The ECG differential diagnosis of AF includes:

- Atrial flutter with variable atrioventricular (AV) conduction where flutter waves may not be clear (obscured).
- Atrial flutter with 2 to 1 AV block.
- Atrial tachycardia with variable AV response.
- Sinus rhythm with frequent atrial premature beats.

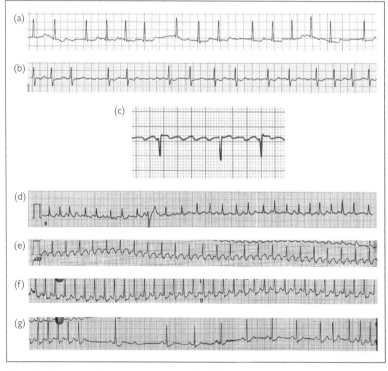

Figure 4.2 Examples of different ECG patterns of AF. (a) Fine AF. (b) Course AF. (c) Lead V₁ (same patient as (b)). (d) AF with rapid ventricular response. (e) Atrial flutter with 2:1 AV conduction. (f) AV nodal re-entrant tachycardia (same patient as (e)). (g) Termination of AVNRT to sinus rhythm with re-initiation of AF (same patient as (f)). See also colour plate section.

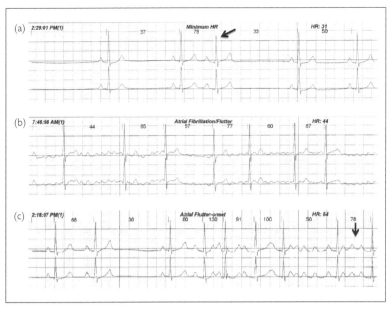

Figure 4.3 Specific ECG patterns of tachy-brady syndrome. (a) Sinus bradycardia with atrial extra-systole (arrow). (b) Atrial fibrillation. (c) Sinus rhythm and atrial flutter (arrow).

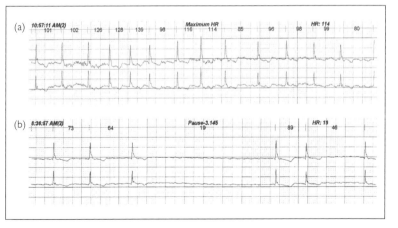

Figure 4.4 ECG patterns from another patient with atrial fibrillation and tachy-brady syndrome. (a) Tachycardia. (b) Bradycardia and pauses.

In such instances, registration of a long rhythm strip and/or multiple leads would provide clues to the correct diagnosis.

An important differential diagnosis is an ECG with a broad QRS morphology, which falls into one of the following categories:

1. If the rhythm is irregular it is AF or atrial flutter, or atrial tachycardia with variable conduction in the presence of established or rate-related right or left bundle branch block. A rare condition is antegrade conduction over an accessory pathway.

2. If the rhythm is regular and the QRS is identical to that during sinus rhythm, it is generally SVT with right or left bundle branch block, or antidromic atrioventricular re-entrant tachycardia (AVRT). In patients with a history of previous myocardial infarction or SHD, a broad QRS tachycardia is usually due to ventricular tachycardia (VT) until proven otherwise. Examination of the AV relationship helps to differentiate supraventricular from ventricular origin. A wide complex tachycardia with different morphologies of sinus rhythm and bundle branch block is always VT.

4.1.2 **Classification of AF**

AF is classified into the following categories based on its duration as shown in Figure 4.5:

1. First-detected or diagnosed AF independent of its duration, and presence or absence of any symptoms.

2. Paroxysmal AF: recurring AF (more than two episodes) lasting less than 24–48 hours that terminate spontaneously but may also last up to 7 days. After this period the rate of spontaneous termination is low and anticoagulation is warranted. Episodes that are longer than 30 seconds are considered recurrence.

3. Persistent AF: episodes lasting longer than 7 days require termination by either direct electrical cardioversion or pharmacological intervention.

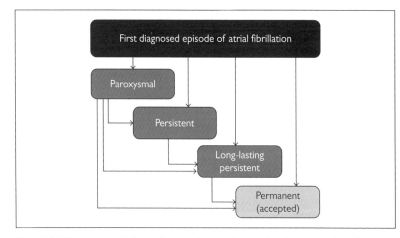

Figure 4.5 Different types of AF according to its duration. Reprinted with permission from Camm AJ, Kirchhof P, Lip GY, Schotten U, Savelieva I, Ernst S, et al. Guidelines for the management of atrial fibrillation: the Task Force for the Management of Atrial Fibrillation of the European Society of Cardiology (ESC). *Europace* 2010; 12:1360–420 by permission of Oxford University Press.

4. Long-lasting persistent AF: episodes lasting longer than 1 year. This definition is created for cases where a rhythm control strategy is recommended mostly to consider catheter ablation of AF.

5. Permanent AF: episodes when patients and their physician accept to maintain AF, or when restoring sinus rhythm is not attempted or failed and rate control is the chosen strategy over rhythm control. Should rhythm management be adopted, the arrhythmia is designed as long-lasting persistent.

6. Lone AF (idiopathic): defined as AF in patients younger than 60 years with no clinically or echocardiographically detectable structural cardiovascular disease, which could be paroxysmal, persistent, or permanent (Potpara et al. 2012 and Wyse et al. 2014).

7. Silent AF (asymptomatic): discovered at routine follow-up or following a complication.

8. Autonomic AF: autonomic nervous system plays an important role in the electrophysiology of the sinus node, atria, and AV node.

   a. Vagal AF: vagaly mediated AF generally occurs in the setting of enhanced parasympathetic tone in paroxysmal forms such as nocturnal AF and after heavy meals. Vagal AF often precedes vomiting, coughing, and the Valsalva manoeuvre, occurring after large meals, diving into cold water, etc. It is usually preceded by sinus bradycardia and/or sinus pauses. The ventricular rate is relatively slow due to the vagal effect on the AV nodal conduction and it is predominantly found in men aged 30–50 years without significant heart disease. Beta-blockers and digoxin may aggravate vagaly mediated AF. Rosso et al. (2010) stated that vagal AF was present in approximately 25% of patients with paroxysmal AF and no SHD. When referred for radiofrequency ablation the procedure was equally effective in both vagal and adrenergic as well as random AF. The prevalence is 6% (Olshansky 2005).

   b. Adrenergic AF: Less common than vagaly mediated AF, and occurs during daytime, provoked by exercise, alcohol, and emotional stress, is often postoperative and is preceded by sinus tachycardia, and polyuria. Ventricular rate is higher during AF and it generally responds well to beta-blockers and/or digoxin. The prevalence is 15% (Olshansky 2005; Rosso et al. 2010).

   (Both vagal and adrenergic AF are often self-terminating.)

4.1.3 Other classifications of AF

Lubitz et al. (2013) recently proposed a simplified classification of AF as follows:

* *AF without 2-year recurrence* was defined as sinus rhythm without any subsequent AF episodes observed after first-detected AF.

* *Recurrent AF* was defined as AF with sinus rhythm of any duration between two AF episodes, including a successful cardioversion.

* *Sustained AF* was defined as the absence of sinus rhythm or successful cardioversion after first-detected AF.

* *Indeterminate patterns* included rhythms other than sinus or AF or those in which a sequence of ECGs included consecutive AF followed by sinus rhythm at the end of the classification window (because AF recurrence could not be verified without examining beyond the classification window).

* *Inadequate data* refers to individuals with only one ECG during the classification window.

Most of these classifications are based on the duration of arrhythmias, symptoms, and detection method; however, they should ideally be disease based so that they can help in the clinical management decision and identify the responders to therapy. The categorization should distinguish between patients on the basis of the severity of the underlying disease, prognosis, clinical symptoms, or indications to therapy (Lubitz et al. 2010a).

4.1.4 **Progression**

AF in younger individuals is usually paroxysmal or persistent and in older individuals becomes more permanent and usually progresses from paroxysmal to permanent. Patients may progress from one category to another depending on the progression of AF. The predictors of progression are not well understood but depend on the development and progression of AF and/or severity of the underlying SHD. Age, diabetes mellitus, and heart failure (HF) are the most important predictors of progression to permanent AF (Pappone et al. 2008).

Although the incidence of AF and progression of AF may share many risk factors, risk factors for progression from paroxysmal to permanent probably mostly depend on worsening of the SHD. A study by Jahangir et al. (2007) on the 30-year follow-up of patients with paroxysmal AF without SHD or hypertension revealed an interesting finding that there was a low risk of progression to permanent AF, contrary to increased mortality, congestive HF, and stroke. The rate of progression from paroxysmal to permanent AF is about 5.5% per year in the Japanese population and 8.6% in the Canadian population (Kato et al. 2004; Kerr et al. 2005, respectively).

ECG recordings during AF episodes are the only way to confirm the diagnosis. ECGs may be normal between the episodes in patients with paroxysmal AF, thus if and when AF is suspected, prolonged ambulatory monitoring can be helpful. After all, some AF patients remain non-progressive despite sharing the same profile and SHD as patients that show progression. Nieuwlaat et al. (2008) reported on a 1-year follow-up of the EuroHeart survey that 46% of the patients with initially first-detected AF episodes did not have AF recurrences, paroxysmal AF patients remained paroxysmal (80%), and 30% of persistent AF patients progressed to permanent and remained permanent (96%).

It should be considered that all of the definitions and classifications mentioned are driven by the patient's perceptions and descriptions of the duration of AF as well as, in part, methods of arrhythmia detection in the patients. An important issue that has recently emerged is the lack of correlation between a patient's symptoms and documented arrhythmias. The clinical relevance of the type of AF and its classification to the clinical management remains a challenge (Lubitz et al. 2010a; Mehall et al. 2007).

4.1.5 **Framingham Risk Score**

The risk score is a gender-specific algorithm used to estimate the 10-year AF risk of an individual and to date the most robust data is from the Framingham Heart Study. A variety of risk factors that are depicted in Figure 4.1 and Table 4.1 such as age, sex, body mass index (BMI), systolic blood pressure, treatment for hypertension, PR interval, clinically significant cardiac murmur, and HF are associated with AF and were incorporated into the risk score model. However, the addition of echocardiographic indices into the risk score model only slightly improved the results. Applying the risk score in primary care could help identify patients at risk of AF and therefore, early detection and intervention targeted to high-risk individuals may be helpful (shown in Table 4.2). Hopefully, by implementation of the risk scores more than half of the AF burden is potentially preventable (Alonso et al. 2013, Benjamin et al. 1998 and 2009). As mentioned by the authors, this data is obtained from white patients and should not be extrapolated to other ethnicities (Lloyd-Jones et al. 2004; Rienstra et al. 2012a.)

4.1.6 **HATCH score**

The HATCH score was developed to identify risk factors that may predict the development of AF from paroxysmal to permanent. It includes hypertension, age (older than 75 years),

Table 4.2 Predicted 10-year risk of atrial fibrillation assigned to the risk score

Risk score	≤0	1	2	3	4	5	6	7	8	9	≥10
Predicted risk	≤1%	2%	2%	3%	4%	6%	8%	12%	16%	22%	>30%

Modified from Schnabel et al., Development of a risk score for atrial fibrillation (Framingham Heart Study): a community based cohort study *Lancet* 2009; 373: 739–45 with permission.

previous transient ischaemic attacks (TIAs) or stroke, chronic obstructive pulmonary disease (COPD), and HF (de Vos et al. 2010; Jahangir et al. 2010). Several longitudinal studies have validated the value of the HATCH score and interestingly the score is not useful in the prediction of the recurrence and progression of AF after catheter ablation (Jahangir et al. 2007).

4.1.7 **Biomarkers**

A biomarker is defined as a characteristic that is objectively measured and evaluated as an indicator of normal biological processes, pathogenic processes, or pharmacological responses to a therapeutic intervention (Biomarkers and Definitions Working Group 2001). Biomarkers are often used to elucidate the pathophysiology of a specific disease and/or to identify individuals at high risk and their response to a specific treatment target. Biomarkers are useful in detecting subclinical diseases, for example, recently B-type natriuretic peptide (BNP) was investigated as a biomarker for incident AF. Data from the Framingham Heart Study stated that the presence of a biomarker panel was associated with an increased risk of AF (Schnabel et al. 2010; Rienstra et al. 2012b). There are a variety of biomarkers related to cardiac injury (myocardial injury), and non-cardiac injury such as markers for coagulation (D-dimer), markers of inflammation (interleukin 6 and C-reactive protein (CRP)), and others such as genetic biomarkers, imaging biomarkers, etc. (Hijazi et al. 2013).

4.1.8 **Clinical presentation in patients with AF**

Clinical presentation in patients with AF is quite variable and mostly dependent on the heart rate and irregularity during AF, underlying SHD, and degree of left ventricular (LV) dysfunction. The symptoms of AF are:

- Palpitation more common in paroxysmal AF, often expressed as racing (and usually irregular) heartbeat.
- Shortness of breath (dyspnoea), exacerbation symptoms of HF.
- Chest pain/chest discomfort.
- Dizziness, light-headedness, and rarely syncope, the latter usually seen in AF with pre-excitation syndrome.
- Diminished exercise capacity, malaise, or fatigue.
- Symptoms of TIA and stroke.
- Impaired quality of life, anxiety, and depression.

The severity of the symptoms depends on the haemodynamic effect of AF (see section on AF and HF). Many patients remain asymptomatic during AF (silent AF) or are asymptomatic between symptomatic episodes. The risk and adverse events in asymptomatic AF patients remain the same or even higher than symptomatic ones (because they are often untreated). On physical examinations the pulse is faster than expected and 'irregularly irregular'. Precipitating causes of episodes such as exercise, emotion, or alcohol need to be identified. Quantification of symptoms such as specific trigger onset, duration, frequency, and severity, are important clinical issues that need to be documented.

4.2 **Atrial fibrillation in conjunction with other arrhythmias**

4.2.1 **AF with profound bradycardia**

Nearly 20% of patients with AF develop profound bradycardia and require permanent pace-maker implantation after reversible causes are excluded (Figure 4.4b). Almost half of these implants are done under urgent hospitalization, even when drug-induced bradycardia has been ruled out. Patients with AF often have episodes of rapid ventricular response followed by bradycardia, the so-called tachy-brady syndrome (Figures 4.3 and 4.4). This condition often requires antiarrhythmic therapy to prevent recurrences of paroxysmal AF and fast heart rate episodes or AV-nodal blocking drugs to control the rapid ventricular rate during AF; the trade-off is a permanent pacemaker implantation. As antiarrhythmic agents are only partially effective, AV nodal ablation with pacemaker implantation is appropriate in a selected group of patients (see Chapter 7). The shortcoming of this approach is that permanent pacemaker implantation which is most often done with right ventricular pacing, creates LV dyssynchrony, a condition that is not desirable since many of these patients have HF (Barrett et al. 2012).

4.2.2 **AF, atrial flutter, and atrial tachycardia**

The coexistence of AF and atrial flutter has been recognized since early investigations of these arrhythmias. In many cases AF precedes atrial flutter and vice versa and sponta-neous transition from one to the other is often observed during long-term monitoring Waldo 2013 (Figure 4.6). Antiarrhythmic therapy often promotes this conversion and its

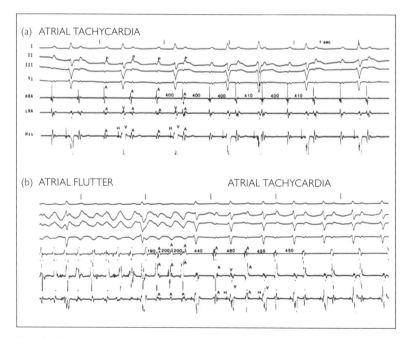

Figure 4.6 Conversion of atrial tachycardia to flutter and back to atrial tachycardia in a patient with paroxysmal AF (not shown here).

effects are often observed prior to conversion to sinus rhythm. Likewise, atrial tachycardia is often present in patients with AF and atrial flutter especially in younger patients with anatomical obstacles such as post-atrial septal defect repair.

4.2.3 AF and atrioventricular nodal re-entrant tachycardia and atrioventricular re-entrant tachycardia

In many cases, it is another type of SVT that is the trigger for AF. Figure 4.7a shows an example of atrioventricular nodal re-entrant tachycardia (AVNRT) transition to AF in a patient with Wolff–Parkinson–White (WPW) syndrome. Figure 4.7b illustrates the transition from AVNRT to AF in a patient with WPW syndrome and broad irregular QRS tachycardia.

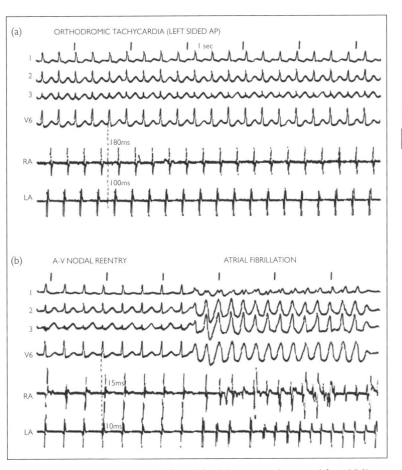

Figure 4.7 (a) Orthodromic tachycardia (AVRT) with left sided accessory pathway, note left atrial (LA) activation precedes the right atrial (RA) activation. (b) atrial ventricular nodal reentrant tachycardia (AVNRT) with short ventriculoatrial conduction, time of 15 ms which converted to AF with conduction over accessory pathway producing irregular wide complex tachycardia typical of patients with AF and WPW syndrome. (c) Conversion of AVRT into AF, note intracardiac electrograms confirm presence of AF.

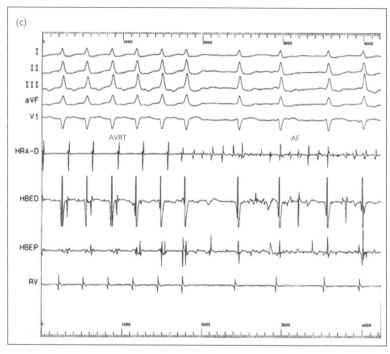

(c)

Figure 4.7 Continued

These findings have significant management implications since ablation of these arrhythmias (AVRT and AVNRT) is feasible with high success rates and will significantly reduce the likelihood of AF in these patient populations.

4.2.4 **AF in patients with WPW syndrome**

It is well established that patients with WPW syndrome carry a higher incidence of AF. AF may occur spontaneously or be triggered by an episode of regular AVRT (Figure 4.7a,b, and c). AF in these patients may occur with very rapid, broad slurred-onset QRS tachycardias with conduction over an accessory pathway that can potentially degenerate to ventricular fibrillation (VF) (Figure 4.8). Obviously, immediate cardioversion is necessary. These patients are often young and have a previous history of palpitations. Careful examination of the ECGs, especially those previous to the event, may point to the correct diagnosis especially if pre-excitation is detected on the ECG. In such cases cardioversion is the safest therapy and medications such as digoxin, calcium antagonists, and lidocaine are contraindicated as they often enhance conduction over the accessory pathway and increase the risk of syncope and/or VF.

4.2.5 **Ventricular arrhythmias in patients with AF**

Patients with AF often have frequent ventricular extrasystoles, couplets, and episodes of non-sustained and sustained VT, especially those with HF and reduced systolic function (Figure 4.9). AF patients with coronary artery disease (CAD) and previous myocardial

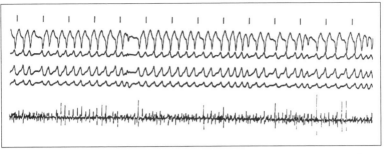

Figure 4.8 An example of AF with rapid irregular wide complex tachycardia. Atrial electrogram (lower panel) confirms the presence of AF. Differential diagnosis is AF in the presence of bundle branch block.

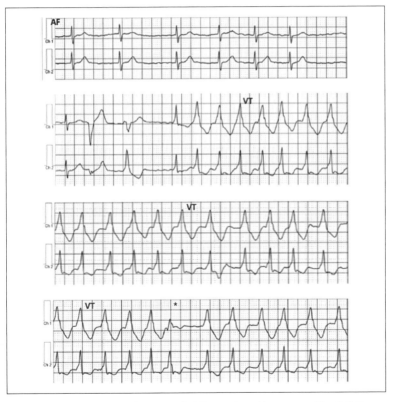

Figure 4.9 An example of sustained monomorphic VT in a patient with permanent AF and HF. Note the VT is initiated after a short–long–short sequence. Star denotes fusion beat.

infarction (LV scar) are at high risk for VT and/or VF, and sudden cardiac death (SCD). In general, the incidence of SCD in patients with AF is more likely than in patients in sinus rhythm. Antiarrhythmic therapy in this cohort is often ineffective and/or carries the risk of proarrhythmia. Management of these cases is a challenge and often requires a multidisciplinary approach, for example, the assistance of both HF and arrhythmia specialists. A hybrid approach is often needed such as implantable cardioverter defibrillator (ICD) or cardiac resynchronization therapy defibrillator (CRT-D) implantation and in selected cases ablation of AF and VT may be considered. (See chapters 5 and 7 for further details).

4.2.6 **Atrial fibrillation and AV block**

In a small number of patients, AF is present in association with complete heart block, usually with junctional escape rhythm with a narrow QRS complex. In cases where the RR interval is very irregular in the presence of AF, one should suspect AF in heart block.

4.3 **Atrial fibrillation and cardiovascular disease**

In general, most patients with early-stage (latent) SHD present with more paroxysmal AF and as the underlying disease progresses, AF also progresses from paroxysmal to persistent and/or permanent. Figure 4.10 illustrates the incidence of types of AF according to their SHD.

4.4 **Atrial fibrillation and hypertension**

Hypertension is the most common cause of AF and is present in 70% of patients with AF. Because of its prevalence, hypertension accounts for more AF than any other risk factor (14%) (Benjamin et al. 1994). Elevated systolic blood pressure (BP), mean arterial BP, and even high normal BP are known risk factors for the development of AF (Grundvold et al. 2012). The risk of AF in patients with hypertension without any other predisposing

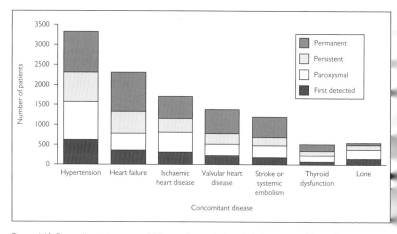

Figure 4.10 Figure illustrates types of AF according to their underlying structural heart disease. Reproduced from Nieuwlaat R, Capucci A, Camm AJ, Olsson SB, Andersen D, Davies DW, *et al.* Atrial fibrillation management: a prospective survey in ESC member countries: the Euro Heart Survey on Atrial Fibrillation. *European Heart Journal* 2005; 26: 2422–34 by permission of Oxford University Press.

factors such as HF, valvular heart disease (VHD), CAD, etc., increases with age and LV mass (Verdecchia et al. 2003). Long-term longitudinal studies from the Framingham Heart Study (Lloyd-Jones et al. 2004) and Women's Health Study revealed that high systolic and diastolic BP increase the risk of developing AF (Tedrow et al. 2010). Pulse pressure is also a recognized risk of new-onset AF (Mitchell et al. 2007). Almost one-third of AF in patients with hypertension remains asymptomatic. A combination of hypertension and AF are present in 72% of stroke patients and 82% of patients with chronic kidney disease, 77% of those with diabetes, 73% of those with CAD, 71% of patients with HF, and 62% of those with metabolic syndrome. In addition, hypertension is seen in 49–90% of AF trials (Manolis et al. 2012) (Figure 4.11).

Hypertensive heart disease is defined as the cardiovascular sequelae of hypertension including left ventricular hypertrophy (LVH), haemodynamic changes (i.e. left atrial enlargement, diastolic dysfunction, and functional mitral regurgitation), and neurohormonal changes. Hypertension increases the likelihood of AF by 40–50% (Raman 2010). LVH is an independent risk factor for AF (Verdecchia et al. 2003). Figure 4.12 demonstrates that there is an increased rate in the incidence of AF in patients with hypertension and LVH as compared with individuals without LVH. Furthermore, new-onset AF in hypertensive patients and those with LVH increases the risk of SCD and stroke independent of other risk factors (Okin et al. 2013). Proarrhythmia related to antiarrhythmic agents or antihypertensive agents particularly those that induce hypokalaemia may play a significant role. Also, development of AF in hypertensive patients may be due to the worsening of underlying SHD that increase the risk of SCD. Although the exact mechanism(s) of the relationship between hypertension and AF is not completely understood, it is believed to be due to the development of atrial hypertrophy, atrial wall stress, and remodelling secondary to renin–angiotensin–aldosterone system activation that induces an inflammatory response, and fibrosis which result in AF (see Figure 4.18 later in chapter). Control of hypertension, particularly

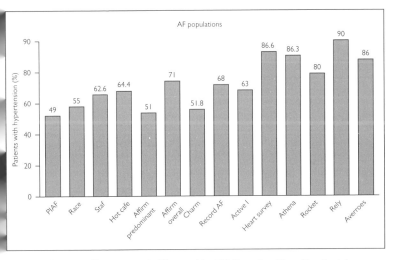

Figure 4.11 Presence of hypertension in different trials of AF. Reproduced from Manolis *et al.*, Hypertension and atrial fibrillation: diagnostic approach, prevention and treatment. Position paper of the Working Group 'Hypertension Arrhythmias and Thrombosis' of the European Society of Hypertension, *Journal of Hypertension* 2011: 30(2): 239–52, with permission from Wolters Kluwer.

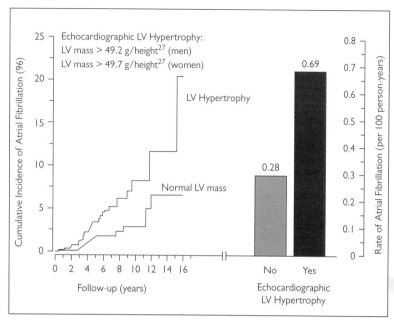

Figure 4.12 Relationship of AF in patients with and without LVH. Reproduced from Verdecchia *et al.*, Atrial Fibrillation in Hypertension: Predictors and Outcome, *Hypertension* 2003; 41(2): 218–23, with permission from Wolters Kluwer.

the reversal (blockade) of the renin–angiotensin–aldosterone system may slow progression of atrial remodelling, fibrosis, and prevent recurrence of AF. Recent meta-analysis of the effect of angiotensin receptor blockers (ARBs) has shown to reduce the incidence of AF and slow its progression to permanent AF. Antihypertensive treatment that is associated with regression of LVH in these patients is associated with lower likelihood of new onset of AF (Okin et al. 2006). On the other hand, another study, the ALLHAT (Antihypertensive and Lipid-Lowering Treatment to Prevent Heart Attack Trial), included therapy such as an angiotensin-converting enzyme (ACE) inhibitor, lisinopril, a dihydropyridine calcium-channel blocker (amlodipine), an alpha-adrenoreceptor blocker (doxazosin), and a thiazide-like diuretic (chlortalidone) to investigate the effects on the incidence of AF. In contrast to the previous reports, the ALLHAT data did not demonstrate significant benefits of antihypertensive therapy on AF and flutter recurrences except for doxazosin (Haywood et al. 2009). Appropriate risk stratification and management should be implemented in lowering the risk of sudden death, HF, and stroke in patients with hypertension and AF.

4.5 **Atrial fibrillation and heart failure**

4.5.1 **AF in HF with diminished LV systolic function (AF and systolic dysfunction)**

AF is the most common arrhythmia in patients with HF, especially in those with reduced systolic function and HF is one of the most common causes of AF (Cha et al. 2004, Havmoller and Chugh 2012, and Savelieva and Camm 2004).

The AF–HF cycle is a complex interaction and relationship between the two diseases (Wongcharoen and Chen 2012). Data from the Framingham Heart Study demonstrated that AF and HF often coexist and that both often have an adverse effect on each other irrespective of which comes first ('chicken or the egg').

The risk of AF and HF after the age of 40 is about 25% and 20% respectively. Data from multiple longitudinal studies suggest AF increases the risk of HF by two- to threefold, and HF also increases the likelihood of AF and promotes AF from paroxysmal to permanent. The Framingham Heart Study demonstrated that at first diagnosis of AF 26% of patients had a history of HF or had concurrent diagnosis of AF. Similarly, at first diagnosis of HF, 24% had previous or concurrent AF. These numbers may be underestimates as the incidence is under-diagnosed due to many cases of asymptomatic AF (Caldwell et al. 2009). As the prevalence of the two diseases increases with age, AF and HF are two important emerging epidemics in medicine (Braunwald 1997 and Olsson et al. 2006). Figure 4.13 illustrates the cumulative incidence of AF in patients with HF (panel a) and the cumulative incidence of HF in patients with AF (panel b). Similar results were reported by Miyasaka et al. (2006). Overall, approximately 40% of individuals with either AF or HF will develop the other condition. Similarly new-onset AF is an independent predictor of in-hospital mortality in patients admitted with HF (Lloyd-Jones et al. 2004; Rivero-Ayerza, et al. 2008; Banerjee et al. 2012). There exists a vicious cycle in which AF begets HF and HF begets AF (Figure 4.14) (Anter et al. 2009).

Haemodynamic consequences of AF: in general, atrial contraction contributes up to 20% of LV stroke volume at rest. The loss of atrial transport (contraction) during AF causes:

- Loss of AV synchrony.
- Irregular heart rate (profound bradycardia or tachycardia.
- Reduction in diastolic LV filling.
- Reduction in stroke volume and cardiac output.
- Decreased LV systolic function (may be related to tachycardia-induced cardiomyopathy).
- An increase in pulmonary artery wedge pressures.
- Increased coronary resistance.

- Impaired myocardial perfusion, especially in patients with coronary artery disease.

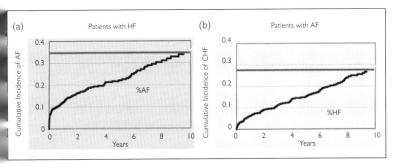

Figure 4.13 (a) Indicates cumulative incidence of HF in patients with AF and (b) indicates cumulative incidence of AF in patients with HF. Reproduced from Wang et al., Temporal Relations of Atrial Fibrillation and Congestive Heart Failure and Their Joint Influence on Mortality: The Framingham Heart Study, *Circulation* 2003; 107(23): 2920–5, with permission from Wolters Kluwer.

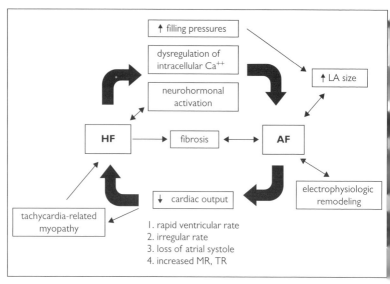

Figure 4.14 The relationship between atrial fibrillation and heart failure. AF: atrial fibrillation; HF: heart failure LA: left atrium; MR: mitral regurgitation; TR: tricuspid regurgitation. Reproduced with permission from Anter et al., Atrial Fibrillation and Heart Failure: Treatment Considerations for a Dual Epidemic, *Circulation* 2009; 119(18): 2516–25 (2009), with permission from Wolters Kluwer.

All of these exert detrimental effects on ventricular function (Rienstra et al. 2012a). Furthermore, an irregular heart rate during AF by itself is associated with reduction in cardiac output when compared with regular sinus rhythm or even ventricular pacing (Clark et al. 1997).

The pathophysiology and cellular mechanisms of AF in HF is beyond the discussion of this review and is well described by (Heist and Ruskin 2006, Morrison et al. 2009, Iwasaki et al. (2011) and Nattel et al. (2007), Nattel et al. (2014)).

AF and HF share common risk factors, mechanisms, and therapeutic strategies. Therefore, optimal management of HF has a beneficial effect on AF progression in addition to restoration of sinus rhythm or at least adequate rate control, which may improve symptoms of HF and delay its progression (Maisel and Stevenson 2003, and Roy et al. 2009). The presence of AF or new-onset AF in patients with HF, either with preserved or reduced systolic function, worsens the quality of life, exercise tolerance, substantially increases the New York Heart Association (NYHA) class of HF, rate of ischaemic stroke, increases frequency of hospitalizations and cost, and often triggers malignant ventricular tachyarrhythmias and SCD (Mountantonakis et al. 2012).

A commonly under-diagnosed entity is AF with uncontrolled ventricular response that promotes development of LV systolic dysfunction now known as 'tachymyopathy' or tachycardia-induced cardiomyopathy. Indeed, this is probably the only type of LV cardiomyopathy that is reversible once the heart rate is controlled. The incidence of tachycardia-induced cardiomyopathy is unknown; however, it has been estimated that in 25–50% of those with LV dysfunction and AF the condition may be related to uncontrolled heart rate (Anter et al. 2009). The severity of the tachymyopathy depends on the heart rate during AF, the duration of AF, and the pre-existing SHD. In patients with no pre-existing SHD, AF-induced tachymyopathy is uncommon and usually after correcting the rate the LV systolic dysfunction returns to normal. In individuals with mild to moderate LV systolic dysfunction, AF-induced tachymyopathy is more common than the former and controlling the heart rate will resume the systolic function to normal or near normal. On the other hand, in patients with severe pre-existing LV dysfunction, the AF-induced tachymyopathy is often under-recognized and correcting the heart rate will partially reverse the tachymyopathy (Cha et al. 2004).

The incidence of AF in patients with HF increases according to the severity of HF and yet remains diverse. Furthermore, the prevalence of AF in HF increases according to the NYHA class ranging from 4% in NYHA class 1 to 50% in NYHA class 4. Data from EuroHeart Failure study that included 10,701 patients hospitalized with HF revealed that 3673 had previous history of AF, 1001 had new-onset AF, and 6027 had no AF. Sudden-onset AF in patients with stable HF may cause acute cardiac decompensation and its severity depends on NYHA functional class. Furthermore, both AF and HF induce neurohormonal changes that contribute to cardiac remodelling. HF also enhances the proarrhythmic effect of AF as well as antiarrhythmic therapy. On the other hand, restoration of sinus rhythm improves cardiac output, exercise capacity, and maximal oxygen consumption.

4.5.2 **AF and diastolic dysfunction (AF with preserved LV systolic function)**

Diastolic dysfunction poses a significant detrimental effect on the atrial structure and function that promotes atrial fibrosis and AF. Unlike AF and LV systolic dysfunction, the pathophysiological relationship between AF and diastolic dysfunction is not well understood and there is a paucity of data on the prevalence of the AF in patients with diastolic dysfunction. The most common findings are left atrial enlargement, increased left atrial afterload and preload, as well as increased atrial wall stress, and fibrosis as promoters of AF (Rosenberg and Manning 2012). Like other aetiologies, hypertension is the most common cause of diastolic dysfunction, followed by LV systolic dysfunction, diabetes, CAD, obesity, and obstructive sleep apnoea (OSA) (McManus et al. 2013). Furthermore, severe diastolic dysfunction is associated with an increased risk of AF. Overall, AF occurs in two-thirds of patients with HF and preserved LV systolic function at some point in their natural history and poses a poor prognosis (Zakeri et al. 2013). Today, the most robust data is from the Cardiovascular Health Study that examined the relationship between diastolic dysfunction and AF in 4480 patients that were followed up for 12.1 years, and AF was documented in 1219 (27.2%) of them. The severity of diastolic dysfunction is an independent determinant that increases the incidence of AF (1% in mild, 12% in moderate, 20% with severe diastolic dysfunction respectively) (Tsang et al. 2002, Jons et al. 2010).

AF also increases the risk of SCD in patients with diastolic dysfunction independently of the other risk factors. The pathophysiological mechanisms and relationship between the diastolic dysfunction and AF is beyond the purpose of this chapter and is well described by Rosenberg and Manning (2012). The management of AF and HF together continues to be a challenge for the practising physician. (See Chapter 5.) The combination of both conditions makes response to therapy and interventions less efficacious. Aggressive interventions should be considered to interrupt the cycle between AF and HF.

4.6 **Atrial fibrillation and coronary artery disease including acute myocardial infarction**

CAD is another major risk factor for AF and increases the risk of AF by four- to fivefold. AF in the setting of chronic CAD and previous myocardial infarction (presence of scar tissue) is a dangerous combination that promotes malignant ventricular arrhythmias and increases the risk of SCD.

AF is a common complication of acute myocardial infarctions (occurring in 6–13% of patients presenting with acute myocardial infarction) and poses an increased risk of morbidity, mortality, prolongs the hospital stay, and may facilitate spontaneous initiation of ventricular tachyarrhythmias. Pedersen et al. (2006) reported that AF and atrial flutter following acute myocardial infarction increase the risk of both sudden and non-sudden cardiovascular death. The combination of CAD and AF also complicates the antithrombotic management strategy for both conditions. AF management with antiarrhythmic therapy in this setting increases the risk of proarrhythmias and SCD. This relationship is further complicated in the setting of acute myocardial infarction. Berton et al. (2009) recently reported on a 7-year follow-up of the adverse effect of AF during acute myocardial infarction. The study comprised 505 patients who were admitted to intensive care units with definite acute myocardial infarction. After adjusting for other co-risk factors, incident AF or atrial flutter was associated with poor prognosis in long-term follow-up, specifically an increased risk of SCD. Management strategies should focus on prevention of AF and atrial flutter in this setting including antiarrhythmic therapy, antithrombotic therapy, and ICD therapy for patients at high risk of SCD. (See Chapter 5.)

4.7 **Atrial fibrillation in patients with valvular heart disease**

Rheumatic VHDs that are associated with AF are mostly mitral stenosis and mitral regurgitation, and prosthetic heart valves. Both rheumatic and non-rheumatic VHDs are significant risk factors for AF. AF increases the risk of stroke by fivefold in non-rheumatic AF and by 17-fold in patients with rheumatic AF (Wachter et al. 2013). Almost 50% of patients with mixed rheumatic mitral valve disease (mitral regurgitation and mitral stenosis) have permanent AF. As the incidence of rheumatic heart disease has declined in Western countries, non-rheumatic valvular disease, mostly mitral regurgitation and aortic valve sclerosis, have become more prevalent. Overall 20% of men and 21% of women with AF have VHD. In general, left-sided VHD especially when associated with left-sided pressure or volume overload, significantly increases the risk of AF. Mitral annular calcification is the most common form of non-rheumatic AF and increases the risk of AF by 1.6-fold.

Patients who undergo transcatheter aortic valve implantation carry a high risk for new-onset AF that adds additional risk for embolic stroke. Approximately one-third of patients without a previous history of AF will develop AF following transcatheter aortic valve implantation. These findings have significant implications both for increased mortality after the procedure as well as antiarrhythmic and antithrombotic management (Amat-Santos et al. 2012).

4.8 **Atrial fibrillation and type 2 diabetes**

Patients with type 2 diabetes are at higher risk of developing new-onset AF compared with age- and gender-matched populations (Nichols et al. 2009). Similarly, patients with type 2 diabetes are at higher risk of progression from paroxysmal to persistent and permanent AF. Overall, diabetes was found in 20% of patients with AF (Aksnes et al. 2008 and Sun and Hu 2010). Huxley et al. (2011) reported on the meta-analysis of the association between diabetes and AF and stated that patients with diabetes had an approximately 40% greater risk of AF compared with those without (relative risk of 1.07–1.6%). This risk rate is relatively high, however, and a rate of 20–25% correlates better with the literature. It should also be noted that the risk of developing AF increases with the duration of diabetes and therefore is time dependent. Patients who had diabetes for more than 10 years demonstrated a higher prevalence of AF (64%) compared with those who had diabetes for less than 5 years (7%) (Du et al. 2009).

The exact mechanism of the relationship between type 2 diabetes and AF is not fully understood. It is, however, thought that it produces cell death as well as inflammation and patchy amyloid in the atrium leading to atrial remodelling, fibrosis, and AF (see Figure 4.18 later in this chapter). One should also consider that type 2 diabetes is often associated with other AF risk factors such as CAD, obesity, insulin resistance, metabolic syndrome, and impaired renal function

4.9 Atrial fibrillation and hypertrophic cardiomyopathy, other cardiomyopathies, pericarditis, and myocarditis

AF is the most common arrhythmia encountered in patients with hypertrophic cardiomyopathy (HCM) with 22% prevalence (Adabag et al. 2005). Patients with HCM carry a four- to sixfold higher risk of AF compared to the general population (Olivotto et al. 2001, Kubo et al. 2009, and Ohe 2009). AF adversely affects the outcome and progression of HCM, and increases the risk of HF and stroke by eightfold in patients with HCM with similar rates between paroxysmal and permanent AF (Maron et al. 2002 and Melacini et al. 2010). It further reflects on the prognosis of HCM and its management strategies such as anticoagulation, antiarrhythmic therapy, and ablative intervention. Left atrial enlargement and fibrosis are also contributing factors to the development of AF in patients with HCM. As the LV compliance is already compromised in these patients, AF will worsen symptoms and reduce exercise tolerance. Similarly, AF appears to be the most significant risk factor in the progression of HF in patients with HCM. In some selected patients, radiofrequency ablation of AF appears appropriate and effective in the management of AF in HCM patients (Di Donna et al. 2010).

4.9.1 Pericarditis and AF

AF may be the first manifestation in patients with acute pericarditis and is often self-terminating. Inflammation plays a significant role in the mechanism and patients with pericarditis respond well to anti-inflammatory medications including colchicine (see Chapter 5).

AF may complicate pericardial effusion and has significant adverse effects in a situation where haemodynamics are already compromised. Like pericarditis, myocarditis may be complicated by AF, which is often self-terminating and often responds to the management of underlying conditions.

4.10 Atrial fibrillation in patients with ischaemic stroke

AF is a major risk factor for stroke and systematic embolization and the risk increases with age (up to five-/sixfold) (Lubitz et al. 2010c). Overall, AF accounts for up to 45% of embolic strokes (75,000–100,000 strokes per year in the United States) (Lloyd-Jones et al. 2010) and the mortality rate is increased especially in women and those with advanced SHD. This in part may be related to a more variable therapeutic range of the international normalized ratio (INR). Stroke risk in AF patients increases in the presence of other co-morbidities such as:

- Advanced age
- Mitral valve disease
- Hypertension

- Peripheral vascular disease
- HF with reduced LV systolic function
- Type II diabetes
- Dyslipidaemia
- Obesity
- Smoking
- Inflammation
- HCM
- Impaired renal function and chronic kidney disease
- Neurohormonal activation (Lubitz et al. 2010b; Jover et al. 2013).

Mediators of stroke in patients with AF include atherosclerotic burden, left atrial dilation and dysfunction, atrial endothelial dysfunction and fibrosis, and a higher hypercoagulable state. Furthermore, AF-related strokes result in more death and disability when compared with strokes due to other causes, since large thrombi may embolize from the left atrium and its appendage to the brain. However, up to 25% of ischaemic strokes in patients with AF may be due to intrinsic cerebrovascular disease and other sources of emboli such as the aorta and carotid arteries. It should be emphasized that the risk of stroke is the same in paroxysmal, persistent, permanent, and symptomatic AF, and that the stroke risk is influenced more by the type of underlying cardiovascular pathology than by the type of AF. AF is part of a broader spectrum of atrial tachyarrhythmias and recent data obtained from implantable devices revealed that atrial tachyarrhythmias in general increase the risk of stroke.

Current guidelines suggest that episodes longer than 6 minutes are significant enough to promote thrombus formation leading to a higher incidence of stroke (Seet et al. 2011). It should be mentioned that the duration of 6 minutes is arbitrarily chosen for trial designs and still remains controversial. These data are further supported by three major trials: MOST, TREND, and ASSERT (Glotzer et al. 2003, 2009; Healy et al. 2012).

4.11 **Asymptomatic 'silent' atrial fibrillation**

Silent AF is defined as AF that occurs in the absence of recognizable symptoms and this is now well established as a risk factor for HF and both silent and manifest stroke. The true incidence of silent AF remains unknown as by its nature it is asymptomatic, thus it may remain undetected (Page 2004). Silent AF is usually found or discovered during routine physical examinations, preoperative workups, or in patients that are admitted with HF, stroke, or other causes. The Stroke Prevention in Atrial Fibrillation Study (SPAF III) data showed that up to 45% of the patients enrolled had ECG documentation of AF (The SPAF III Writing Committee for the Stroke Prevention in Atrial Fibrillation Investigators 1998). It is estimated that more than 50% of patients with AF have asymptomatic AF episodes and the risk and complications of asymptomatic AF, particularly stroke and HF, are indeed similar or higher than symptomatic AF. One study reported 12 times as many asymptomatic as symptomatic AF in 38% of patients with implanted pacemakers and even episodes longer than 48 hours of AF were asymptomatic. The majority of these patients were not on anticoagulation agents. In symptomatic AF often there is little correlation between symptoms and rhythms. The Canadian Registry of AF study showed that 21% of patients with AF were asymptomatic (Kerr et al. 2005).

Furthermore in patients that undergo AF ablation for symptomatic AF, asymptomatic episodes may occur after the procedure. Therefore the symptom-based success rate of catheter and surgical ablation of AF may overestimate the success rate of the procedure

(Hindricks et al. 2005). Interestingly, the incidence of detected asymptomatic AF increases after AF ablation. Verma et al. (2013) reported in a prospective multicentre study on the incidence of asymptomatic and symptomatic episodes of AF before and after ablation and found that the ratio of episodes increased from 1.1 to 1.7 after ablation. They extended their conclusion that symptoms alone underestimate post-ablation burden with 12% of the patients having asymptomatic recurrences.

4.11.1 **AF and silent stroke**

AF was found in about 25% of patients admitted with ischaemic stroke. The recent data from the Atrial Fibrillation Follow-up Investigation of Rhythm Management (AFFIRM) follow-up suggests that up to 57% of strokes occurred in those patients who assumed that AF was suppressed (A Comparison of Rate Control and Rhythm Control in Patients with Atrial Fibrillation 2002). Overall it is estimated that the risk of stroke is sixfold higher in asymptomatic than symptomatic AF patients.

Recently, two important trials elaborated on the significance of asymptomatic AF and other atrial arrhythmias on the risk of stroke (ASSERT trial) (Healy et al. 2012). The data was obtained from patients who had either a pacemaker or ICD; 2580 patients with hypertension were enrolled, aged 65 years or older with no history of documented AF. The primary outcome was ischaemic stroke or systemic embolisms. The study revealed that subclinical (asymptomatic) atrial arrhythmias occurred frequently in patients with a pacemaker or ICD and were associated with a significant 2.5-fold increase in risk of stroke or systemic embolism (Figure 4.15). The other trial (TRENDS) provided similar data and conclusions (Glotzer et al. 2009). These findings have significant therapeutic implications for both AF and stroke management. Similar concerns are now emerging in patients with AF who undergo pulmonary vein ablation, in whom a high incidence of asymptomatic AF is reported and a high incidence of subclinical cerebral embolism is detected (Gaita et al. 2010).

Early investigations using Holter monitoring reported about a 3% incidence of AF in cryptogenic stroke. However, with modern devices such as implantable loop recorders where monitoring can be expanded to weeks or months, the detection of AF in this population is increasing up to 50%. The annual rate of embolic events in patients with bradycardia is reported to be between 6% and 10% and the annual incidence of ischaemic stroke in patients with pacemakers and sinus node disease has been reported to be around 1% to 1.4% (Capucci et al. 2005). Continuous monitoring appears to be superior to intermittent recording, particularly when the effectiveness of AF treatment and procedures are being evaluated. Modern implantable pacemakers and ICDs with accurate diagnostic algorithms and large storage capacity provide an excellent opportunity for evaluation and management of cardiac arrhythmias.

In summary, it appears that silent AF and stroke are often related. Therefore screening for one could potentially detect the other. This was well investigated in a report by Friberg et al. (2013) in the STROKESTOP trial and Sanna et al. (2014).

4.12 **Atrial fibrillation and cognition**

Recent investigations suggest that AF is independently associated with decreased cognition and dementia. Alzheimer's disease is the most common dementia in the elderly and accounts for 60–80% of cases (Bunch et al. 2010). Risk factors for dementia are advanced age, diabetes, hypertension, smoking, HF, stroke, and systemic inflammation and are almost the same in risk factors for AF. However, multivariable analysis demonstrates that AF is indeed an independent risk factor for developing all forms of dementia. A study by Bunch et al. (2010) surprisingly revealed risk of cognitive impairment and related conditions were higher in younger AF patients. Individuals with AF have an adjusted twofold increased risk of

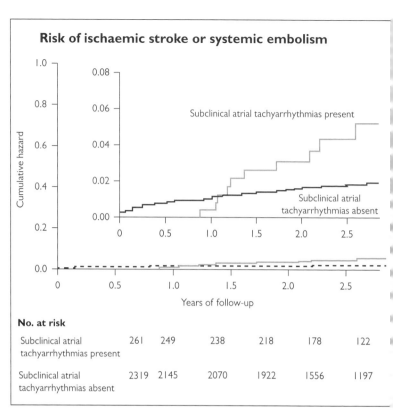

Risk of ischaemic stroke or systemic embolism

Figure 4.15 Demonstrates incidence of subclinical stroke in patients with and without subclinical atrial tachyarrhythmias. Reproduced with permission from Healy *et al.*, Subclinical atrial fibrillation and the risk of stroke. *N Engl J Med* 2012; 366: 120–9.

dementia. Presence of silent brain infarcts on magnetic resonance imaging (MRI) independent of its aetiology doubles the risk of dementia and such findings may identify individuals at a high risk (Vermeer et al. 2003). Currently, however, there is no data to suggest that early intervention in AF would lower the risk of dementia.

4.13 **Atrial fibrillation and sleep apnoea, obesity, and metabolic syndrome**

Obstructive sleep apnoea (OSA), defined as abnormal apnoea–hypopnoea index of more than ten episodes per hour of sleep, is a recognized independent risk factor for AF. Approximately two-thirds of patients with paroxysmal or persistent AF have suffered from OSA. In general, OSA is more prevalent in middle-aged men, than women, 25% and 9% respectively (Belhassen 2013). OSA significantly increases incident AF independently of its other related aetiologies (Figure 4.16). A similar study showed that nearly half of the patients with AF had OSA. The exact mechanism and relationship between OSA and AF is not fully

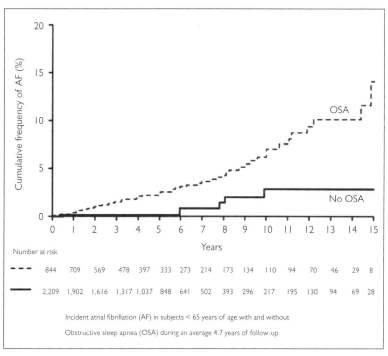

Incident atrial fibrillation (AF) in subjects < 65 years of age with and without

Obstructive sleep apnea (OSA) during an average 4.7 years of follow-up

Figure 4.16 Incidence of AF in patients < 65 years of age with and without OSA during an average of 4–7 years of follow up. Reproduced with permission from Caples et al., Sleep disordered breathing and atrial fibrillation. *Prog Cardiovasc Dis* 2009; 51(5): 411–15.

understood. It is suggested that (1) periodic hypoxia and hypercapnia, (2) intrathoracic pressure oscillations, (3) an increase in sympathetic surge, (4) increased oxidative stress, (Li et al. 2010) (5) diastolic dysfunction leading to fibrosis, and (6) increased cardiac chamber enlargement predispose to AF (Monahan et al. 2009). Like other pathologies, OSA and AF share many common risk factors. The detailed pathophysiology of OSA and its relationship with AF and other cardiovascular diseases is described in Jaffe et al. (2013) and Dimitri et al. (2012). OSA increases the occurrence rate of AF after cardioversion and catheter ablation as well as lowering the response rate of AF to antiarrhythmic therapy (Chilukuri et al. 2010, and Tang et al. 2009). This effect is more evident in patients with severe OSA. Treatment of OSA with continuous positive airways pressure may improve AF ablation success, and lowers the recurrence rate (Patel et al. 2010). Fein et al. (2013) recently reported that treatment of OSA might reduce the risk of AF recurrence after catheter ablation. Screening for OSA in patients with AF who are candidates for cardioversion and AF ablation may be considered.

4.13.1 **AF, metabolic syndrome, and obesity**

Metabolic syndrome is described by the presence of central obesity, atherogenic dyslipidaemia, hypertension, insulin resistance, low high-density lipoprotein cholesterol, proinflammatory state, prothrombotic state, and hyper-tryglyceridaemia (Grundy et al. 2004).

Although obesity is a part of metabolic syndrome, by itself it is a risk factor for the incidence of AF. Patients with obesity have up to a 2.4-fold increased AF risk (Conen 2013).

This when compared to non-obese individuals makes for about a 40–50% increased risk of developing AF (Magnani et al. 2013). Tsang et al. (2008) and Abed and Wittert (2013) reported a follow-up of up to 21 years and found that obesity is an independent risk factor for progression of paroxysmal to permanent AF independent of BMI and left atrial volume. Furthermore, as hypertension, adult-onset diabetes (type 2 diabetes), and diastolic dysfunction are common in obesity, they also increase the risk of AF. Obese subjects with a BMI of 25–30 kg/m^2 had a 35% likelihood of developing AF, whereas those with BMI of more than 30 kg/m^2 had up to a 78% risk of developing AF (Zhuang et al. 2013). High BMI values are an independent predictor of increased left atrial size, and subsequently AF. Similarly, data from the Women's Health Study showed each 1-unit increase in BMI was associated with a 4.7% increase in the risk of developing AF. Interestingly those women who reduced their BMI to < 30 kg/m^2 had a reduced risk of AF. OSA and obesity are modifiable risk factors and interventions to promote normal weight may reduce the risk of AF and its burden (Wang et al. 2004). Both OSA and obesity are associated with increased inflammatory markers that in turn produce atrial fibrosis and cardiac remodelling leading to AF (Drager et al. 2013 and Karasoy et al. 2013).

Obesity and metabolic syndrome share many risk profiles for AF as other causes described in Table 4.1. The mechanisms and pathogenesis by which metabolic syndrome and obesity promote AF are unclear but in part may be related to the development of left atrial enlargement, LV diastolic dysfunction, inflammation, fibrosis, and endothelial dysfunction Figure 4.17 illustrates potential mechanisms involved in the association of obesity, metabolic syndrome, and AF. Patients with AF associated with metabolic syndrome demonstrate a lower response to antiarrhythmic therapy as well as catheter ablation procedures and cardioversion. Therefore, physicians should inform patients about the relationship between obesity and AF as well as the potential benefit of interventions to reduce their BMI and subsequently lower the risk of AF.

4.14 **Atrial fibrillation and other medical conditions**

Hyperthyroidism, whether overt or subclinical (defined as reduced serum thyroid stimulating hormone (TSH) concentration but with normal rage of free thyroxin level), causes AF. It is estimated that about 10–15% of patients with hyperthyroidism develop AF during the course of their disease. In patients with subclinical hyperthyroidism the risk of AF is three to five times higher than control patients. The prevalence of subclinical thyroid dysfunction is high and it is underdiagnosed since the symptoms are often mild (Selmer et al. 2012). Patients with thyrotoxicosis are at the highest risk of AF and often present with rapid ventricular response, and urgent management may be required.

Overt hypothyroidism (increased TSH with normal free thyroxin levels) is common in the adult population and is associated with bradycardia and blunted heart rate response to exercise and both overt and subclinical hypothyroidism is associated with a lower risk of AF

Amiodarone is widely used for management of patients with AF. Chronic use of amiodarone may cause both hypothyroid and hyperthyroid dysfunction and the latter may then increase the risk of AF. Discontinuation of amiodarone may resolve the problem, but antithyroid medication is often needed. Interval thyroid function testing is recommended in patients under chronic amiodarone therapy.

4.14.1 **AF and kidney disease**

There is increasing evidence of an association between chronic kidney disease and AF. Chronic kidney disease may be found in about 35% of patients with AF (Capodanno and Angiolillo 2012 and Winkelmayer 2013). The relationship between the two diseases is expected to increase and is underestimated as they share many risk profiles, including

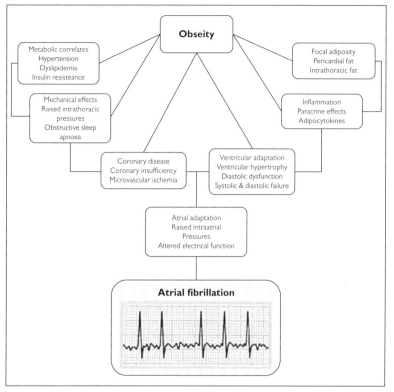

Figure 4.17 The predominant intermediate mechanisms, including clinical pathways and atrial remodelling, that bridge obesity and atrial fibrillation. Reproduced with permission from Magnani et al., Obesity begets atrial fibrillation: a contemporary summary Circulation 2013; 123: 401–5.

hypertension, diabetes, HF, and age (Baber et al. 2011). There is a linear relationship between degree of impaired renal function and the risk of developing new-onset AF (Watanabe et al. 2009). Bansal et al. (2013) recently reported that incident AF is independently associated with increased risk of progression of chronic kidney disease towards developing end-stage renal disease.

Patients in end-stage renal disease and those treated with renal dialysis are at the highest risk for the development of AF ranging from 10% to 17%. Newly diagnosed AF doubles mortality in patients with end-stage renal disease who are on dialysis. Similarly, recent onset of AF in older patients initiating renal dialysis increases the mortality rate by 50% during the first year (Goldstein et al. 2012). New-onset and persistent AF in post-kidney transplant patients is associated with poor outcome (Lenihan et al. 2013). This association further affects the prognosis and complicates management of AF in these patients who need antiarrhythmic and novel antithrombotic agents (Capodanno and Angiolillo 2012 and Nimmo et al. 2013). Therefore it is recommended that patients receiving antithrombotic therapy should be screened for chronic kidney disease and often dose adjustment may be needed under those conditions (Piccini et al. 2013, Camm and Savelieva 2013, Marinigh et al. 2011, and Olesen et al. 2012).

4.14.2 **AF in pulmonary disease**

Acute pulmonary embolism may be complicated by sudden-onset AF (in about 10% of cases), often with a rapid ventricular response. AF in this situation may resolve spontaneously.

Patients with long-standing COPD often suffer from a variety of atrial arrhythmias including AF and atrial flutter, recurrent chronic obstructive pulmonary disease, atrial tachycardia, and multifocal atrial tachycardia (the latter being more common). These arrhythmias often persist and management is challenging as many medications require cautious use or are contraindicated in this situation.

4.14.3 **AF in patients with peripheral vascular disease**

The association of peripheral vascular disease (PVD) and AF was less appreciated until recently. Suffice to say the recent European Society of Cardiology 2010 guidelines on the management of patients with AF included PVD on its risk stratification score CHA_2DS_2-VASc (congestive HF or LV dysfunction, hypertension, age $\geq$ 75 years, diabetes, vascular disease (PVD, myocardial infarction, aortic plaque), sex category (female gender)). PVD was present in 8% of AF patients who were non-smokers and in 14% of AF those who were smokers.

4.14.4 **Medication-induced AF**

Alpha-agonist medications and other sympathomimetic drugs are underdiagnosed causes of AF precipitations with rapid ventricular response. Careful medication review with patients helps to identify these causes.

Patients who receive adenosine for termination of SVTs may transiently develop AF.

Intravenous bisphosphonate therapy in cancer patients has been reported by rare incidence of AF and stroke, however conflicting results are available regarding oral bisphosphonates and the risk of AF and flutter in women (Wilkinson et al. 2010, and Gross et al. 2009 respectively; Loke et al. 2009).

4.14.5 **AF in congenital heart disease**

Patients with congenital heart disease may present with AF at some point in the course of their disease. Atrial septal defect is the most common congenital heart disease associated with AF and flutter. Patients with post-atrial septal defect repair and those with any form of surgery involving atriotomy may present with this arrhythmia after a few years. AF in this setting is often associated with other arrhythmias, specifically atrial tachycardia or atrial flutter. Radiofrequency ablation of atrial flutter and tachycardia is very effective and also decreases the incidence of AF.

4.15 **Atrial fibrillation during endurance exercise and competitive sports (athletes)**

In general, moderate exercise and physical activity have a beneficial effect on the cardiovascular system. Light to moderate exercise, specifically walking, is generally accepted as safe and, if anything, lowers the incidence of AF. On the other hand, extreme (vigorous) exercise and competitive activities may have deleterious effects. AF is the most common form of arrhythmias in athletes at about 5–10%, that is, about fivefold normal (Calvo et al. 2012). The incidence varies according to the type of sport activity. The highest rates are among marathon runners, cyclists, and cross-country skiers. AF in this setting generally occurs after prolonged, high-intensity activity. Interestingly with detraining, these physiological cardiac changes reverse and therefore the incidence of sports-related AF decreases, although left atrial dilation does not completely reverse. It is important to note, however, that detraining is virtually an impossible treatment strategy. Cardiac remodelling including atrial and ventricular dilation, inflammatory changes, fibrosis, and increased vagal tone are among potential mechanisms of exercise-induced AF (McClaskey et al. 2013). Increased vagal tone is a common physiological response to prolonged vigorous exercise and by itself is not enough to promote AF. Another possible connection between sports and AF is the usage of anabolic steroids as there has been evidence found on athletes developing AF after the use of such substances (Schoonderwoerd et al. 2008).

4.16 Atrial fibrillation and alcohol, caffeine use, recreational drugs, and smoking

4.16.1 AF and alcohol

The association between alcohol consumption and AF has been long recognized and AF is the most common arrhythmia related to ethanol abuse (Kodama et al. 2011 and Mukamal et al. 2005). Alcohol consumption is known to increase the risk of AF in a dose-dependent fashion. Acute alcohol overdose also provokes sudden-onset AF, the so-called holiday heart syndrome, defined as acute cardiac rhythm and/or conduction disturbances associated with heavy ethanol consumption in a person without other clinical evidence of heart disease and disappearing with abstinence without evident residual (Ettinger et al. 1978). Several mechanisms for alcohol-induced AF have been proposed: (1) increasing adrenergic tone and decreasing vagal tone; (2) direct effect on atrial and ventricular myocardium; (3) chronic alcohol use causing dilated cardiomyopathy (alcoholic cardiomyopathy) and increasing the risk of AF; (4) an increase in intra-atrial conduction time and P-wave duration which is also a risk factor for AF; (5) association of alcohol abuse with other co-morbidities such as hypertension diabetes, HF, and obesity; and (6) low socioeconomic profile. In a study by Schoonderwoerd et al. (2008) it was found that when the amount of alcohol consumed equated to more than 36 g per day or about three drinks per day the risk of developing AF is increased by 34%. Consumption of 35 or more drinks per week among men is associated with a 1.5-fold increase in AF after adjusting for other risk factors. It is, however, important to distinguish alcohol-induced vaso-vagal response from ethanol toxicity.

4.16.2 AF and caffeine

It is the general belief that as a stimulant, caffeine may cause palpitations and increase the risk of cardiac arrhythmias. However, several large population studies have revealed that regular caffeine use does not increase the risk of AF. A large study by Frost and Vestergaard (2005) examined the effect of coffee and other caffeinated drinks on AF and atrial flutter among participants with an average age of 56 years and followed up for 5.7 years. The result of this study demonstrated that the moderate consumption of coffee was not associated with an increased risk of AF or atrial flutter (Frost and Vestergaard 2005). Likewise, Conen et al. (2010a) examined the effects of coffee consumption on the incidence of AF in women. Healthy women participated in the Women's Health Study who were of 45 years of age and above, were free of cardiovascular disease, and were followed for 14.4 years. The results showed that in this large cohort of initially healthy women, coffee consumption did not increase the risk of AF. Two recent publications in 2013 further elaborated the benefits of habitual (mild to moderate) coffee consumption and specifically none of the reports indicated the increased risk of atrial arrhythmias. Needless to say large amounts of coffee may produce occasional palpitations, anxiety, tremors, insomnia as well as bone loss (O'Keefe et al. 2013). Caffeine toxicity by self-intended poisoning produces supraventricular and ventricular tachyarrhythmias.

Caldeira et al. (2013), in a meta-analysis study, reported that caffeine does not increase the risk of AF.

4.16.3 **AF and recreational drugs**

Recreational substances (illicit drugs) can potentially be arrhythmogenic. The most commonly used is cannabis (marijuana) with its cardiovascular effects including sinus tachycardia and vasovagal syncope. This usually is seen in individuals under the age of 45. Cannabis-induced AF is rare and is often self-terminating, and apart from abstinence there are no specific guidelines for its management (Krishnamoorthy et al. 2009).

Another recreational drug that is commonly used and potentially may induce AF is cocaine. It is a potent sympathomimetic, stimulating adrenergic receptors that increase the heart rate and enhance vasoconstriction. With its direct effect on the atrial myocardium it can potentially provoke AF (Krishnamoorthy et al. 2009).

4.16.4 **AF and smoking**

Smoking is a known risk factor in increasing the risk of AF. Meta-analysis and the data from the Atherosclerosis Risk in Communities (ARIC) demonstrated that smoking is associated with increased risk of AF by more than twofold (Chamberlain et al. 2011). Interestingly, there is a trend towards a lower incidence of AF among smokers who have quit smoking.

4.17 **Postoperative atrial fibrillation**

4.17.1 **AF in post-cardiac surgery**

AF is the most common arrhythmia after cardiac surgery and occurs in approximately 20–50% of patients depending on the type of surgery, specifically in 30–40% of patients post coronary artery bypass graft (CABG), up to 60–70% of patients with combined CABG and valve surgery, and in 11–24% of patients after cardiac transplantation (Helgadottir et al. 2012). Sixty per cent of the episodes occur on day 2–3 of post-op and 57% of the patients experience only one episode (Kaw et al. 2011). The majority of the post-op AF converts to sinus rhythm in the first 24–48 hours and if it takes longer than 48 hours there is an increased risk of stroke. AF in post-cardiac surgery may cause HF and haemodynamic instability, and may prolong hospital stays, increasing costs by 20%. (Refer to Table 4.3 for predictors of intra-, pre-, and postoperative AF.) Postoperative AF affects both early and late mortality after isolated CABG surgery. Most of the complications are related to stroke therefore careful postoperative surveillance for antithrombotic prophylaxis is warranted (Mariscalco et al. 2008). Post pericardiotomy and inflammation play a significant role in the pathophysiology of post-cardiac surgery AF (Echahidi et al. 2008).

Management of patients after cardiac surgery should focus on preoperative risk profiling to identify those who are at a high risk and who are eligible for prophylactic treatment according to the guidelines (Rho 2009). Rader et al. (2011) reported that white patients had a higher marked risk of postoperative AF than black and other non-Caucasian patients (Matthew et al. 2004, and Omae and Kanmura 2012).

4.17.2 **AF after non-cardiac surgery**

Likewise, major non-cardiac surgery poses an increased risk of AF with similar consequences such as prolonged hospitalization and increased cost. Similar appropriate management applies.

Table 4.3 A summary of the risk factors for preoperative, intraoperative, and postoperative AF		
Preoperative	**Intraoperative**	**Postoperative**
Age, male gender, race	Damage to the atrium	Volume overload
Previous history of AF	Atrial ischemia/infarction	Increased after load
HF	Acute volume change	Hypertension/hypotension
Previous cardiac surgery	Insertion of a ventilator tube	Inflammation
Concomitant valve surgery	Venous cannulation	Atrial extrasystole
LV dysfunction	Electrolyte imbalance	Post-pericardiotomy syndrome
Renal dysfunction	Systolic BP > 180 mm or < 80 mm	Autonomic nervous system imbalance
Hypertension	Inadequate cardiac protection during bypass	Electrolyte imbalance
Diabetes	Hyperadrenergic state	Post-op anaemia
Valvular heart disease	Right coronary artery surgery, etc.	Longer duration of mechanical ventilation
Obesity/metabolic syndrome	Atriotomy	Pericarditis/pericardial effusion
High BNP levels		
Stroke		
Previous MI		
COPD		
LA size and volume		
Pre-op β-blockers		
Withdrawal of β-blockers		
P wave duration > 116 ms		
BNP = b-type natriuretic peptide; BP = blood pressure; COPD = chronic obstructive pulmonary disease; HF = heart failure; LA = left atrium; LV = left ventricular; MI = myocardial infarction.		

4.18 **Atrial fibrillation and sudden cardiac death**

AF per se is known to increase the risk of SCD independently of other cardiovascular risk factors. The Framingham Heart Study reported that AF increases the risk of death by 1.5-fold in men and 1.9-fold in women. A similar finding was also reported in studies by Miyasaka et al. (2007) as well as Chen et al. (2013). The mechanism of this increased mortality is not fully understood but the possible contributing factors include:

- Reduced LV systolic performance due to irregular heart rate, particularly in a short–long–short manner in patients with previous myocardial infarction (scar tissue) that facilitate limitation of ventricular tachyarrhythmias.
- Fast heart rate during AF, which promotes tachycardia-induced cardiomyopathy.

- Repolarization abnormalities and QT prolongation due to LV remodelling and increased sympathetic activity that may cause malignant ventricular arrhythmia and proarrhythmic effects of antiarrhythmic therapy

Recognition of this association is important and provides opportunities to reduce the risk of SCD in patients with AF as well as appropriate therapy including antiarrhythmic and antithrombotic agents that are discussed in other chapters.

4.19 **Genetics of atrial fibrillation**

There is now compelling evidence that genetics play an important role in different types of AF and AF is part of a spectrum of monogenic cardiac diseases such as HCM, Brugada syndrome, long QT syndrome, sodium channel mutations, and sinus node dysfunction. Genetic heterogeneity appears to be a prominent feature of all inherited arrhythmias. The most common type of genetic AF is linked to chromosome 4q25 (Kaab et al. 2009). In addition, to date several genes have been identified including *KCNQ1, KCNE2, KCNE5, GJA5, SCN5A, SCN1B/2B,* and *NPPA* and more are being discovered that cause the development of AF. Moreover, multiple mutations can cause various forms of genetically related AF and have been described in families with autosomal dominant AF in the genes listed previously. Genome-wide association studies have identified common genetic variance associated with AF (Magnani et al. 2011). However, at present genetic testing is not recommended and has no prognostic or therapeutic impact in patients with familial AF (Fatkin et al. 2007; Lubitz et al. 2010b; Ackerman et al. 2011). Specific forms of genetically related AF are familial AF, and AF in inherited channelopathies as described (Everett et al. 2013). Only 5% of patients with AF are known to have disease-associated genes. For further information see the Heart Rhythm Society and European Heart Rhythm Associations expert consensus statement on the state of genetic testing for channelopathies and cardiomyopathies (Ackerman et al. 2011).

4.20 **Familial atrial fibrillation and atrial fibrillation in inherited channelopathies**

Lone AF is defined as AF occurring in patients aged 60 years or younger in the absence of overt SHD and is often associated with other inherited channelopathies. Lone AF accounts for 3–11% of all AF patients, and some reported up to 30% (Menezes et al. 2013).

First-degree relatives of individuals with AF, especially those with no SHD, are at greater risk of developing AF (Zoller et al. 2012). Data from the Framingham Heart Study revealed that 27% of patients with AF had a first-degree relative with AF. Also, the risk of AF is increased by 40% in those patients with familial AF irrespective of other risk factors. A report by Lubitz et al. (2010d) demonstrated a close relationship between familial AF and new-onset AF. Christophersen et al. (2013) reported a 20% increase in mortality rate from familial AF in twins who had a co-twin with AF. The implication of this finding suggests that the discovery of AF in a young patient should result in the screening of his/her siblings.

Specific genes and their chromosomal locations have been identified. Cardiac sodium channel mutations have been demonstrated in patients with familial AF, Brugada syndrome, long and short QT syndromes, as well as other inherited arrhythmias. It is recommended that first-degree family members of individuals with familial and lone AF be investigated for the presence or history of AF. Smith et al. (2013) recently reported an interesting finding on the genetic association of AF and HF in a large population study and concluded the presence of a heritable component to the presence of AF in patients with HF. Over the past decade several inherited cardiac diseases and channelopathies have been recognized to be associated with

AF. A large population study by Nielsen et al. (2013) reported an interesting finding that both short and long QT intervals were associated with higher incidents of lone AF.

4.20.1 Brugada syndrome and AF

Brugada syndrome is another example of a genetic disease characterized by ST segment elevation in precordial leads V1–V3 (Brugada type ECG) and propensity to life-threatening ventricular arrhythmias and SCD (Junttila et al. 2008). Aside from its risk of SCD and ventricular tachyarrhythmias, AF is the most common arrhythmia in Brugada syndrome patients (approximately 20%). Francis and Antzelevitch (2008) reported a review of the literature on the incidence of AF and Brugada syndrome, which ranged from 6% to as high as 100%. Interestingly, most AF has occurred in Brugada type I ECG pattern (Bigi et al. 2007). Indeed, Rodríguez-Mañero et al. (2013) reported on a large group of 611 patients with Brugada syndrome and found that 35% had AF before the Brugada syndrome was diagnosed and that AF may be the first manifestation of the concealed Brugada syndrome. It was also reported that AF is associated with the increased risk of arrhythmic events in patients with Brugada syndrome (Kusano et al. 2008). Itoh et al. (2001) reported on the arrhythmias in patients with Brugada-type ECG findings in 30 patients and interestingly found ventricular fibrillation in nine out of the 30 patients as well as AF in nine out of the 30 patients. These findings have significant implications such as the initiation of antiarrhythmic as well as anticoagulation/ antithrombotic therapy. Class IC antiarrhythmic agents may increase the risk of sudden death in patients with Brugada syndrome (Postema et al. 2009). Atrial arrhythmias in Brugada syndrome further increase the risk of inappropriate ICD shocks (Francis and Antzelevitch 2008). The mechanism of this high prevalence of AF in patients with Brugada syndrome remains speculative.

4.20.2 AF and short and long QT syndrome

Patients with short and long QT syndrome beside their risk of ventricular arrhythmias and SCD have a high prevalence of AF. A significant improvement in the understanding of the genetic substrate underlying AF improves the detection of not only affected individuals but also their relatives that are at high risk. Recent studies suggest that these inherited channelopathies may share common genetic factors or mutations (Pizzale et al. 2008). For example, *SCN5A* mutations in AF are associated with other inherited arrhythmias (Darbar et al. 2008). Similarly, AF has been reported to coexist in patients with catecholaminergic polymorphic VT. One can foresee that in the future the role of genetic testing will be more implemented in genotype-guided determination of a patient's natural history of morbidity-related AF with other SHDs such as hypertension, dementia, etc. Genotype-guided management strategies, and efficacy prediction, will result in significantly better preventive strategies (Lubitz et al. 2010d). Since the genes have now been identified for familial AF and other related channelopathies, recognition of such cases in clinic and genetic counselling should be considered. Appropriate management including screening and antithrombotic and antiarrhythmic therapy is warranted.

4.21 Atrial fibrillation during pregnancy and in postmenopausal women

AF is rare during pregnancy, especially in patients without a history of AF. However, in patients with a previous history of AF, pregnancy may increase the risk of AF. Postpartum cardiomyopathy is also associated with an increased risk of AF. The risk of AF increases during the postmenopausal period irrespective of other risk factors (Magnani et al. 2012).

4.22 **Atrial fibrillation, inflammation, and fibrosis**

Relationship between inflammation and cardiovascular disease has long been recognized, from as early as the 1920s. AF is clearly associated with increased level of inflammatory markers (Guo et al. 2012). Several biomarkers of inflammation in patients with AF have been identified (Table 4.1) and CRP was found (in non-postoperative AF) to be elevated in patients with AF (Conen et al. 2010b, and Lappegard et al. 2013).

Atrial biopsies in patients with AF have also confirmed the presence of inflammation (Boldt et al. 2004). There is also evidence supporting a link between inflammation, fibrosis, and AF, and some of the drug therapies, such as the ACE-inhibitors, ARBs, steroids, fish oils, and vitamin C, that might be efficacious in the prevention of AF by modulating inflammatory pathways. Virtually all aetiologies of AF cause inflammation, fibrosis, and remodelling (electrical, mechanical, structural, and neurohormonal) which promote AF. Figure 4.18 illustrates inflammation and fibrosis as final common pathways that lead to AF. As fibrosis plays a significant role in the perpetuation and maintenance of AF, innovative, preventative, and therapeutic strategies besides reversal of underlying SHDs should focus on the prevention of inflammation, fibrosis, and remodelling or at least reverse remodelling (Velagapudi et al. 2013).

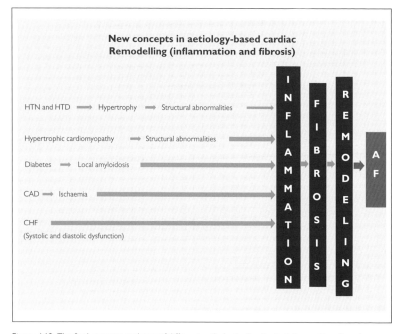

Figure 4.18 The final common pathway of different pathologies leading to inflammation, fibrosis, remodelling, and AF. Innovative interventions beside the targeted underlying structural heart diseases should focus on prevention of inflammation and fibrosis. With permission from Shenasa et al., Individualized therapy in patients with atrial fibrillation: new look at atrial fibrillation *Europace* 2012; 14: v121–4.

4.23 **Atrial fibrillation detected in patients with implantable devices**

Implantable devices provide a unique opportunity to investigate the natural history and response to antiarrhythmic and ablative procedures in patients with AF and a variety of other arrhythmias as well as trial designs. AF detected from implantable devices increases the risk of embolic stroke by 3.1-fold when lasting more than 24 hours (Zimetbaum and Goldman 2010). New-onset AF in patients with ICD and CRT-D/pacemaker (P) increases the risk of inappropriate shock and adversely affects the long-term outcome. Furthermore, even with new devices with advanced algorithms, AF in patients with implantable devices can still cause inappropriate shock and increase mortality. The use of antiarrhythmic therapy to control AF often has adverse effects as many patients suffer from HF and are at risk of proarrhythmia. Detection of AF and atrial flutter in these patients warrants anticoagulation and antithrombotic therapy as well as carefully selected antiarrhythmic therapy. Figure 4.19 illustrates an example of atrial arrhythmia detected at the time of routine device interrogation while the patient denied any symptoms.

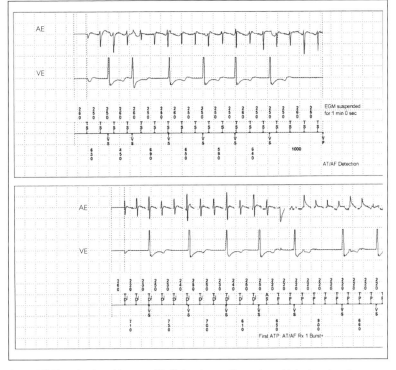

Figure 4.19 Example of atrial flutter and fibrillation detected in a patient with implanted cardioverter defibrillator who reported no symptoms. The top VE panel depicts the atrial electrogram and the lower panel depicts ventricular electrogram AE.

4.24 **Atrial fibrillation in cardiac resynchronization therapy patients**

CRT is now an established therapy in patients with HF, LV dyssynchrony, left bundle branch block, and QRS duration ≥ 120 ms, and reduced LV ejection fraction (30% or less). As discussed earlier, AF is very common in patients with HF. Current data suggests that AF impacts the response to CRT, and new-onset AF in these patients has had adverse effects on CRT response as well as on long-term outcome. Borleffs et al. (2010 and 2009) reported that 25% of recipients of CRT without previous history of AF developed new-onset AF during follow up (32 ± 15 months) and those patients demonstrated less favourable responses to CRT (i.e. less LV reverse remodelling and less event-free courses). On the other hand, conflicting results are available on the effect of CRT on the incidence of AF. The current trend is that CRT lowers the incidence of AF, although no prospective studies are available (Hoppe et al. 2006).

4.25 **Diagnostic tools and screening for atrial fibrillation and their limitations**

Figure 4.20 depicts different monitoring devices that are currently available.
Heart rhythm monitoring is indicated for the following purposes:

* Assessing treatment efficacy for rate or rhythm control.
* Evaluating safety and efficacy of antiarrhythmic drug therapy and ablative procedures.
* Finding the correlation between documented arrhythmias and symptoms.
* Monitoring for AF burden to determine stroke risk (Camm et al. 2010 and Capucci et al. 2005).

ECG remains the main, at least first, diagnostic test in patients with AF. However, in patients with paroxysmal AF and those with asymptomatic AF, the ECG is of limited value and is often of a 'hit or miss' nature. The diagnostic yield of ECG to detect new AF is only 1% whereas intermittent ECG recording yields only 7%. Furthermore, the 12-lead ECG reflects the resting heart rate during AF and does not provide information on activity-related or nocturnal patterns of AF. In the analysis of the ECG, markers of other electrical abnormalities such as PR and QRS prolongation, long or short QT intervals, Brugada syndrome, and pre-excitation syndrome (presence of a delta wave), and other electrical abnormalities need to be carefully examined. Similarly, markers of non-electrical disease such as hypertrophy, cardiomyopathies, hypertension, and remote or acute myocardial infarction also need to be identified. Figure 4.21 compares the diagnostic yield of different monitoring systems.

As the significance of silent AF is increasingly recognized, the need for more accurate detection and characterization by devices is imminent. The technical detailed description of these devices can be found in the paper by Mittal et al. (2011).

4.25.1 **Holter monitoring**

Holter monitoring is commonly used in patients with a history of palpitations, syncope, near syncope, or suspected arrhythmias. The diagnostic yield of Holter monitoring in patients with undocumented AF is also low (7%). Engdahl et al. (2013) reported a stepwise screening of AF in a 75-year-old population in Sweden. They included patients who at entry were in sinus rhythm with no history of AF and a $CHAD_2S$ risk score ≥ 2. Patients were given a handheld ECG reader and asked to read 20–30 seconds twice daily and also if palpitations occurred. One per cent of the population was diagnosed with newly detected persistent AF, 7% with paroxysmal AF, 9% of the participants were candidates for oral anticoagulation,

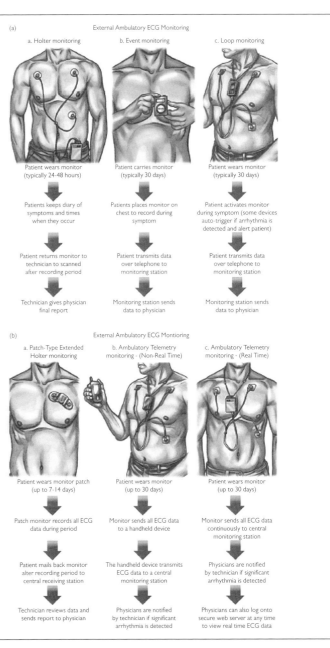

(a)   External Ambulatory ECG Monitoring

a. Holter monitoring   b. Event monitoring   c. Loop monitoring

Patient wears monitor (typically 24-48 hours) → Patient carries monitor (typically 30 days) → Patient wears monitor (typically 30 days)

Patients keeps diary of symptoms and times when they occur → Patient places monitor on chest to record during symptom → Patient activates monitor during symptom (some devices auto-trigger if arrhythmia is detected and alert patient)

Patient returns monitor to technician to scanned after recording period → Patient transmits data over telephone to monitoring station → Patient transmits data over telephone to monitoring station

Technician gives physician final report → Monitoring station sends data to physician → Monitoring station sends data to physician

(b)   External Ambulatory ECG Montioring

a. Patch-Type Extended Holter monitoring   b. Ambulatory Telemetry monitoring - (Non-Real Time)   c. Ambulatory Telemetry monitoring - (Real Time)

Patient wears monitor patch (up to 7-14 days) → Patient wears monitor (up to 30 days) → Patient wears monitor (up to 30 days)

Patch monitor records all ECG data during period → Monitor sends all ECG data to a handheld device → Monitor sends all ECG data continuously to central monitoring station

Patient mails back monitor alter recording period to central receiving station → The handheld device transmits ECG data to a central monitoring station → Physicians are notified by technician if significant arrhythmia is detected

Technician reviews data and sends report to physician → Physicians are notified by technician if significant arrhythmia is detected → Physicians can also log onto secure web server at any time to view real time ECG data

Figure 4.20 (a) Demonstrates different external rhythm monitoring devices. Reproduced with permission from Mittal et al., Ambulatory external electroardiographic monitoring; focus on atrial fibrillation *J Am Coll Cardiol* 2011; 58: 1741–9. (b) Demonstrates a leadless arrhythmia monitoring device that is placed as a patch over the torso. Courtesy of iRhythm, with permission.

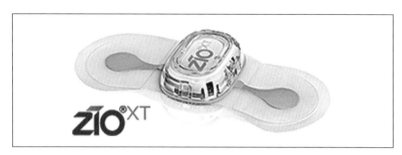

Figure 4.20 Continued

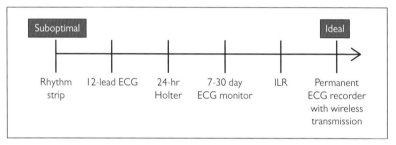

Figure 4.21 Spectrum of ambulatory ECG monitoring modalities. As one moves from the left to right the duration of monitoring increases which in turn increases the diagnostic yield. ILR: implantable loop recorder. Reproduced with permission from Mittal *et al.*, Ambulatory external electroardiographic monitoring; focus on atrial fibrillation *J Am Coll Cardiol* 2011; 58: 1741–9.

and almost 50% of the patients with known AF were not on anticoagulation (Engdahl et al. 2013). Another report from the same group showed that this stepwise screening proved to be cost-effective (Friberg et al. 2010).

4.25.2 External loop recorders

External loop recorders and event monitors provide 16–18% diagnostic yield, increasing up to 50% with the use of ambulatory cardiac telemetry and new cellular technology.

4.25.3 Implantable devices

Apart from pacemakers and ICDs that provide nearly 90–100% accurate diagnostic yield with the rate and timing of the events, implantable loop recorders provide important information in patients suspected of cardiac arrhythmias, syncope, stroke, and post-ablation follow-up. However, this data is from a very highly selected patient group that already had such devices. Hindricks et al. (2010) reported that the overall accuracy of an implantable leadless cardiac monitor is 98.5% in patients with AF. Overall, there is a significantly higher detection of recurrent paroxysmal AF with implanted devices compared to ECG recordings (device: 88%, ECG: 46%, P < 0.0001) (Israel et al. 2004).

The new era of digital monitoring via smart phones has opened a new window for the detection of a variety of arrhythmias with instant report to the physicians. This probably will

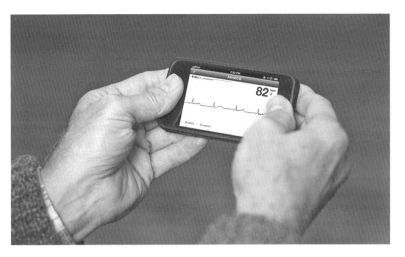

Figure 4.22 AliveCor® handheld heart monitoring device on a smart phone. Courtesy of AliveCor® with permission.

be the future of detecting arrhythmias and immediate intervention if needed. Figure 4.22 shows one example of a handheld device that is integrated in a smart phone and the rhythms can be captured and emailed to the healthcare providers using the device. The limitation of this device, however, is that patients record the rhythm randomly or only when they have symptoms thus asymptomatic events may be missed.

The cost of the approved ambulatory ECG monitoring according to the Medicare Reimbursement Fee Schedule are as follows:

- Holter monitor: US$236.85
- External event monitors (up to 30 days): US$631.27
- Mobile cardiovascular telemetry: US$889.30
- Implantable loop devices: US$1000.00.

4.26 Forecasting the future of atrial fibrillation

AF is a very complex arrhythmia in terms of its evolving epidemiology, multiple and diverse aetiologies, progression, co-morbidities, and complications as well as socioeconomic burden. After a century of progress, AF management remains unsatisfactory and challenging. This is in part due to the parallel intricate relationship of aging and evolving SHD and association with all-cause and cardiac mortality. AF should no longer be regarded as a single entity and diagnostic and therapeutic approaches should consider its genetic profile, and specific aetiology, in an evidence-based personalized approach. With the available technology, early detection of even the preclinical phase of the disease and its related aetiologies as well as a better understanding of its natural history should be mandatory (Wang 2011). Team management including virtual telemedicine in partnership with multidisciplinary involvement such as primary care, general cardiologist, rhythmologist, and paramedical assistance is the way to the future (please see the proposal by Berti et al. (2013)).

The risk markers of AF are too non-specific and physicians are faced with a large number of patients that need to be treated in order to lower the risk. Better recognition of genetic profiles and pharmacogenetics may help identify the higher-risk patients and responders and eliminate excessive treatment.

References

A Comparison of Rate Control and Rhythm Control in Patients with Atrial Fibrillation (2002). The Atrial Fibrillation Follow-up Investigation of Rhythm Management (AFFIRM) Investigators. *N Engl J Med* 347(23): 1825–33

Abed HS, Wittert GA (2013). Obesity and atrial fibrillation. *Obes Rev* 14(11): 929–38.

Ackerman MJ, Priori SG, Willems S, Berul C, Brugada R, Calkins H, *et al.* (2011). HRS/EHRA Expert consensus statement on the state of genetic testing for the channelopathies and cardiomyopathies. *Europace* 13: 1077–109.

Adabag AS, Casey SA, Kuskowski MA, Zenovich AG, Marjon BJ (2005). Spectrum and prognostic significance of arrhythmias on ambulatory Holter electrocardiogram in hypertrophic cardiomyopathy. *J Am Coll Cardiol* 45: 687–704.

Aksnes TA, Schmieder RE, Kjeldsen SE, Ghani S, Hua TA, Julius S (2008). Impact of new-onset diabetes mellitus on development of atrial fibrillation and heart failure in high-risk hypertension (from the VALUE trial). *Am J Cardiol* 101: 634–8.

Alonso A, Krijthe BP, Aspelund T, Stepas KA, Pencina MJ, Moser CB, *et al.* (2013). Simple risk model predicts incidence of atrial fibrillation in a racially and geographically diverse population: the CHARGE-AF consortium. *J Am Heart Assoc* 2: e000102.

Amat-Santos IJ, Rodes-Cabau J, Urena M, DeLarochelliere R, Doyle D, *et al.* (2012). Incidence, predictive factors and prognostic value of new-onset atrial fibrillation following transcatheter aortic valve implantation. *J Am Coll Cardiol* 59: 178–88.

Anter E, Jessup M, Callans DJ (2009). Atrial fibrillation and heart failure: treatment considerations for a dual epidemic. *Circulation* 119: 2516–25.

Baber U, Howard VJ, Halperin JL, Soliman E, Zhang X, McClellan W, *et al.* (2011). Association of chronic kidney disease with atrial fibrillation among adults in the United States: REasons for Geographic and Racial Differences in Stroke (REGARDS) Study. *Circ Arrhythm Electrophysiol* 4: 26–32.

Banerjee A, Taillandier S, Olesen JB, Lane DA, Lallemand B, Lip GYH, *et al.* (2012). Ejection fraction and outcomes in patients with atrial fibrillation and heart failure: the Loire Valley Atrial Fibrillation Project. *Eur J Heart Fail* 14: 295–301.

Bansal N, Fan D, Hsu C, Ordonez JD, Marcus GM, Go AS (2013). Incident atrial fibrillation and risk of end-stage renal disease in adults with chronic kidney disease. *Circulation* 127: 569–74.

Barrett TW, Abraham RL, Jenkins CA, Russ S, Storrow AB, Darbar D (2012). Risk factors for bradycardia requiring pacemaker implantation in patients with atrial fibrillation. *Am J Cardiol* 110: 1315–21.

Belhassen B (2013). Continuous positive airway pressure after circumferential pulmonary vein isolation. *J Am Coll Cardiol* 62(4): 306–7.

Benjamin EJ, Chen PS, Bild DE, Mascette AM, Albert CM, Alonso A, *et al.* (2009). Prevention of atrial fibrillation: report from a national heart, lung and blood institute workshop. *Circulation* 119: 606–18.

Benjamin EJ, Levy D, Vazisiri SM, D'Agostino RB, Belanger AJ, Wolf PA (1994). Independent risk factors for atrial fibrillation in a population-based cohort: the Framingham Heart Study. *JAMA* 271: 840–4.

Benjamin EJ, Wolf PA, D'Agostino RB, Silbershatz H, Kannel WB, Levy D (1998). Impact of atrial fibrillation on the risk of death: the Framingham Heart Study. *Circulation* 98: 946–52.

Berti D, Hindriks JML, Brandes A, Deaton C, Crijns HJGM, Camm AJ, *et al.* (2013). A proposal for interdisciplinary nurse-coordinated atrial fibrillation expert programmes as a way to structure daily practice. *Eur Heart J* 34: 2725–30.

Berton G, Cordiano R, Cucchini F, Cavuto F, Pellegrinet M, Palatini P (2009). Atrial fibrillation during acute myocardial infarction: association with all-cause mortality and sudden death after 7-year follow up. *Int J Clin Pract* 63: 712–21.

Bigi MA, Aslani A, Shahrzad S (2007). Clinical predictors of atrial fibrillation in Brugada syndrome. *Europace* 9: 947–50.

Biomarkers and Definitions Working Group (2011). Biomarkers and surrogate endpoints: preferred definitions and conceptual framework. *Clin Pharmacol Ther* 69(3): 89–95.

Boldt A, Wetzel U, Lauschke J, Weigl J, Gummert J, Hindricks G, *et al.* (2004). Fibrosis in left atrial tissue of patients with atrial fibrillation with and without underlying mitral valve disease. *Heart* 90: 400–5.

Borleffs CJW, van Rees JB, van Welsenes GH, van der Velde ET, van Erven L, Bax JJ, *et al.* (2010). Prognostic importance of atrial fibrillation in implantable cardioverter-defibrillator patients. *J Am Coll Cardiol* 55: 879–85.

Borleffs CJW, Ypenburg C, van Bommel RJ, Delgado V, van Erven L, Schalij MJ, *et al.* (2009). Clinical importance of new onset atrial fibrillation after cardiac resynchronization therapy. *Heart Rhythm* 6: 305–10.

Braunwald E (1997). Shattuck lecture—cardiovascular medicine at the turn of the millennium: triumphs, concerns, and opportunities. *New Engl J Med* 337(19): 1360–9.

Bunch TJ, Weiss P, Crandall BG, May HT, Bair TL, Osborn JS, *et al.* (2010). Atrial fibrillation is independently associated with senile vascular, and Alzheimer's dementia. *Heart Rhythm* 7: 433–7.

Caldeira D, Martins C, Alves LB, Pereira H, Ferreira JJ, Costa J. (2013). Caffeine does not increase the risk of atrial fibrillation: a systematic review and meta-analysis of observational studies. *Heart* 99: 1383–9.

Caldwell JC, Contractor H, Petkar S, Ali R, Clark B, Neyses L, *et al.* (2009). Atrial fibrillation is under-recognized in chronic heart failure: insights from a heart failure cohort treated with cardiac resynchronization therapy. *Europace* 11: 1295–300.

Calvo N, Brugada J, Sitges M, Mont L (2012). Atrial fibrillation and atrial flutter in athletes. *Br J Sports Med* 46: i37–43.

Camm JA, Kirchhof P, Lip GYH, Schotten U, Savelieva I, Ernst S, *et al.* (2010). Guidelines for the management of atrial fibrillation. *Eur Heart J* 31: 2369–429.

Camm JA, Savelieva I (2013). "R" is for "Renal" and for "Risk": refining risk stratification for stroke in atrial fibrillation. *Circulation* 127: 169–71.

Caples SM, Somers VK (2009). Sleep-disordered breathing and atrial fibrillation. *Prog Cardiovasc Dis* 51(5): 411–15.

Capodanno D, Angiolillo DJ (2012). Antithrombotic therapy in patients with chronic kidney disease. *Circulation* 125: 2649–61.

Capucci A, Santini M, Padeletti L, Gulizia M, Botto G, Boriani G, *et al.* (2005). Monitored atrial fibrillation duration predicts arterial embolic events in patients suffering from bradycardia and atrial fibrillation implanted with antitachycardia pacemakers. *J Am Coll Cardiol* 46: 1913–20.

Cha YM, Redfield MM, Shen WK, Gersh BJ (2004). Atrial fibrillation and ventricular dysfunction: a vicious electromechanical cycle. *Circulation* 109: 2839–43.

Chamberlain AM, Agarwal SK, Folsom AR, Duval S, Soliman EZ, Ambrose M, *et al.* (2011). Smoking and incidence of atrial fibrillation: results from the Atherosclerosis Risk in Communities (ARIC) Study. *Heart Rhythm* 8: 1160–6.

Chen LY, Sotoodehnia N, Buzkova P, Lopez FL, Yee LM, Heckbert SR, *et al.* (2013). Atrial fibrillation and the risk of sudden cardiac death: the Atherosclerosis Risk in Communities Study and Cardiovascular Health Study. *JAMA* 173(1): 29–35.

Chin LY, Shen Win-Kuang (2007). Epidemiology of atrial fibrillation: a current perspective. *Heart Rhythm* 4: S1–6.

Chilukuri K, Dalal D, Gadrey S (2010). A prospective study evaluating the role of obesity and obstructive sleep apnea for outcomes after catheter ablation of atrial fibrillation. *J Cardiovasc Electrophysiol* 21: 521–5.

Christophersen IE, Budtz-Jorgensen E, Olesen MS, Haunso S, Christensen K, Svendsen JH (2013). Familial atrial fibrillation predicts increased risk of mortality: a study in Danish twins. *Circ Arrhythm Electrophysiol* 6: 10–15.

Chung MK, Martin DO, Sprecher D, Wazni O, Kanderian A, Carnes CA, *et al.* (2001). C-reactive protein elevation in patients with atrial arrhythmias inflammatory mechanisms and persistence of atrial fibrillation. *Circulation* 104: 2886–91.

Clark DM, Plumb VJ, Epstein AE, Kay GN. (1997). Hemodynamic effects of an irregular sequence of ventricular cycle lengths during atrial fibrillation. *J Am Coll Cardiol* 30: 1039–45.

Conen D (2013). Obesity and atrial fibrillation: the evidence is gaining weight. *Europace* 15: 771–2.

Conen D, Chae CU, Glynn RJ, Tedrow UB, Everett BM, Burning JE, *et al.* (2011). Risk of death and cardiovascular events in initially healthy women with new-onset atrial fibrillation. *JAMA* 305: 2080–7.

Conen D, Chiuve SE, Everett BM, Zhang SM, Buring JE, Albert CM (2010a). Caffeine consumption and incident atrial fibrillation in women. *Am J Clin Nutr* 92: 509–14.

Conen D, Ridker PM, Everett BM, Tedrow UB, Rose L, Cook NR, *et al.* (2010b). A multimarker approach to assess the influence of inflammation on the incidence of atrial fibrillation in women. *Eur Heart J* 31: 1730–6.

Darbar D, Kannankeril PJ, Donahue BS, Kucera G, Stubblefield T, Haines JL, *et al.* (2008). Cardiac sodium channel (SCN5A) variants associated with atrial fibrillation. *Circulation* 117: 1927–35.

De Souza AI, Camm AJ (2012). Proteomics of atrial fibrillation. *Circ Arrhythm Electrophysiol* 5: 1036–43.

De Vos CB, Pisters R, Nieuwlaat R, Prins MH, Tieleman RG, Coelen RJS, *et al.* (2010). Progression from paroxysmal to persistent atrial fibrillation: clinical correlates and prognosis. *J Am Coll Cardiol* 55: 725–31.

Dimitri H, Ng M, Brooks AG, Kuklik P, Stiles MK, Lau DH, *et al.* (2012). Atrial remodeling in obstructive sleep apnea: implications for atrial fibrillation. *Heart Rhythm* 9(3): 321–7.

Di Donna P, Olivotto I, Delcre SDL, Caponi D, Scaglione M, Nault I, *et al.* (2010). Efficacy of catheter ablation for atrial fibrillation in hypertrophic cardiomyopathy: impact of age, atrial remodeling, and disease progression. *Europace* 12: 347–55.

Drager LF, Togeiro SM, Polotsky VY, Lorenzi-Filho G (2013). Obstructive sleep apnea: a cardiometabolic risk in obesity and the metabolic syndrome. *J Am Coll Cardiol* 62: 569–76.

Du X, Ninomiya T, de Galan B, Abadi E, Chalmers J, Pillai A, *et al.* (2009). Risks of cardiovascular events and effects of routine blood pressure lowering among patients with type 2 diabetes and atrial fibrillation: results of the ADVANCE study. *Eur Heart J* 30: 1128–35.

Echahidi N, Pibarot P, O'Hara G, Mathieu P (2008). Mechanisms, prevention, and treatment of atrial fibrillation after cardiac surgery. *J Am Coll Cardiol* 51: 793–801.

Engdahl J, Andersson L, Mirskaya M, Rosenqvist M (2013). Stepwise screening for atrial fibrillation in a 75-year-old population: implications for stroke prevention. *Circulation* 127: 930–70.

Ettinger PO, Wu CF, De La Cruz C, Weisse AB, Ahmed SS, Regan TJ (1978). Arrhythmias and the "Holiday Heart": alcohol associated cardiac rhythm disorders. *Am Heart J* 95: 555–62.

Everett BM, Cook NR, Conen D, Chasman DI, Ridker PM, Christine AM (2013). Novel genetic markers improve measures of atrial fibrillation risk prediction. *Eur Heart J* 34: 2234–51.

Fatkin D, Otway R, Vandenberg JI (2007). Genes and atrial fibrillation: a new look at an old problem. *Circulation* 116: 782–92.

Fein AS, Shvilkin A, Shah D, Haffajee CI, Das S, Kumar K, *et al.* (2013). Treatment of obstructive sleep apnea reduces the risk of atrial fibrillation recurrence after catheter ablation. *J Am Coll Cardiol* 62: 300–5.

Francis J, Antzelevitch C (2008). Atrial fibrillation and Brugada syndrome. *J Am Coll Cardiol* 51: 1149–53.

Friberg L, Engdahl J, Fykman v, Svennberg E, Levin J, Rosenqvist M (2013). Population screening of 75- and 76-year-old men and women for silent atrial fibrillation (STROKESTOP). *Europace* 15: 135–40.

Friberg L, Hammar N, Rosenqvist M (2010). Stroke in paroxysmal atrial fibrillation: report from the Stockholm Cohort of Atrial Fibrillation. *Eur Heart J* 31: 967–75.

Frost L, Vestergaard P (2005). Caffeine and risk of atrial fibrillation or flutter: the Danish Diet, Cancer, and Health Study. *Am J Clin Nutr* 81: 578–82.

Fye BW (2006). Tracing atrial fibrillation – 100 years. *N Engl J Med* 355(14): 1412–14.

Gaita F, Caponi D, Pianelli M, Scaglione M, Toso E, Cesarani F, *et al.* (2010). Radiofrequency catheter ablation of atrial fibrillation: a cause of silent thromboembolism? Magnetic resonance imaging assessment of cerebral thromboembolism in patients undergoing ablation of atrial fibrillation. *Circulation* 122: 1667–73.

Glotzer TV, Daoud EG, Wyse G, Singer DE, Ezekowitz MD, Hilker C, *et al.* (2009). The relationship between daily atrial tachyarrhythmia burden from implantable device diagnostics and stroke risk: the TRENDS Study. *Circ Arrhythmia Electrophysiol* 2: 474–80.

Glotzer TV, Hellkamp AS, Zimmerman J, Sweeney MO, Yee R, Marinchak R, *et al.* (2003). Atrial high rate episodes detected by pacemaker diagnostics predict death and stroke: report of the Atrial Diagnostics Ancillary Study of the Mode Selection Trial (MOST). *Circulation* 107: 1614–19.

Go AS, Hylek EM, Philips KA, Chang Y, Henault LE, Selby JV, et al. (2001). Prevalence of diagnosed atrial fibrillation in adults: national implications for rhythm management and stroke prevention: the AnTicoagulation and Risk Factors in Atrial Fibrillation (ATRIA) Study. JAMA 285(18): 2370–5.

Go AS, Mozaffarian D, Roger VL, Benjamin EL, Berry JD, Border WB, et al. (2013). Heart disease and stroke statistics- 2013 update: a report from the American Heart Association. 127: e6–245.

Goldstein BA, Arce CM, Hlatky MA, Turakhia M, Setoguchi S, Winkelmayer WC (2012). Trends in the incidence of atrial fibrillation in older patients initiating dialysis in the United States. Circulation 126: 2293–301

Gross A, Douglas I, Hingorani A, MacAllister R, Smeeth L (2009). Oral bisphosphonates and risk of atrial fibrillation and flutter in women: a self-controlled case-series safety analysis. Plos One 4(3): e4720.

Grundvold I, Skretteberg PT, Liestol K, Erikssen G, Kjeldsen SE, Arnesen H, et al. (2012). Epidemiology/population science: Upper normal blood pressures predict incident atrial fibrillation in healthy middle aged men. Hypertension 59: 198–204

Grundy SM, Brewer HB, Cleeman JI, Smith SC, Lenfant C (2004). Definition of metabolic syndrome: report of the National heart, Lung, and Blood Institute/American Heart Association Conference on Scientific Issues Related to Defintion. Circulation 109: 433–8.

Guo Y, Lip GYH, Apostoakis S (2012). Inflammation in atrial fibrillation. J Am Coll Cardiol 60: 2263–70.

Havmöller R, Chugh SS (2012). Atrial fibrillation in heart failure. Curr Heart Fail Rep 9: 309–18.

Haywood LJ, Ford CE, Crow RS, Davis BR, Massie BM, Einhorn PT, et al. (2009). Atrial fibrillation at baseline and during follow-up in ALLHAT (Antihypertensive and Lipid-Lowering Treatment to Prevent Heart Attack Trial. J Am Coll Cardiol 54: 2023–31

Healy JS, Connolly SJ, Gold MR, Israel CW, Van Gelder IC, Capucci A, et al. (2012). Subclinical atrial fibrillation and the risk of stroke. N Engl J Med 366: 120–9.

Heist EK, Ruskin JN (2006). Atrial fibrillation and congestive heart failure: risk factor, mechanisms, and treatment. Prog Cardiovasc Dis 48(4): 256–69.

Helgadottir S, Sigurdsson MI, Ingvarsdottir IL, Arnar DO, Gudbjartsson T (2012). Atrial fibrillation following cardiac surgery: risk analysis and long-term survival. J Cardiothorac Surg 7: 87.

Hess PL, Kim S, Piccini JP, Allen LA, Ansell JE, Chang P, et al. (2013). Use of evidence-based cardiac prevention therapy among outpatients with atrial fibrillation. Am J Med 126: 625–32.

Hijazi Z, Oldgren J, Siegbahn A, Granger CB, Wallentin L (2013). Biomarkers in atrial fibrillation: a clinical review. Eur Heart J 34(20): 1475–80.

Hindricks G, Piorkowski C, Tanner H, Kobza R, Gerds-Li JH, Carbucicchio C, et al. (2005). Perception of atrial fibrillation before and after radiofrequency catheter ablation relevance of asymptomatic arrhythmia recurrence. Circulation 112: 307–13.

Hindricks G, Pokushalov E, Urban L, Taborsky M, Kuck KH, Lebedev D, et al. (2010). Performance of a new leadless implantable cardiac monitor in detecting and quantifying atrial fibrillation results of the XPECT trial. Circ Arrhythm Electrophysiol 3: 141–7.

Hoppe UC, Casares JM, Eiskjaer H, Hagemann A, Cleland JG, Freemantle N, et al. (2006). Effect of cardiac resynchronization on the incidence of atrial fibrillation in patients with severe heart failure. Circulation 114: 18–25.

Huxley RR, Fillion KB, Alonso A (2011). Meta-analysis of cohort and case-control studies of type 2-diabetes mellitus and risk of atrial fibrillation. Am J Cardiol 108(1): 56–62.

Israel CW, Gronefeld G, Ehrlich JR, Li YG, Hohnloser SH (2004). Long term risk of recurrent atrial fibrillation as documented by an implantable monitoring device: implications for optimal patient care. J Am Coll Cardiol 43(1): 47–52.

Itoh H, Shimizu M, Ino H, Okeie K, Yamaguchi M, Fujino N, et al. (2001). Arrhythmias in patients with Brugada-type electrocardiographic findings. Jpn Circ J 65: 483–6.

Iwasaki Y, Nishida K, Kato T, Nattel S. (2011). Atrial fibrillation pathophysiology. Circulation 123: 2264–74.

Jaffe LM, Kjekshus J, Gottlieb SS (2013). Importance and management of chronic sleep apnoea in cardiology. Eur Heart J 34: 809–15.

Jahangir A, Murarka S (2010). Progression of paroxysmal to persistent atrial fibrillation. J Am Coll Cardiol 55(8): 732–4.

Jahangir A, Lee V, Friedman PA, Trusty JM, Hodge DO, Jahangir A, et al. (2007). Long- term progression and outcomes with aging in patients with Lone atrial fibrillation: a 30 year follow up study. *Circulation* 115: 3050–6.

Jons C, Joergensen RM, Hassager C, Gang UJ, Dixen U, Johannesen A, et al. (2010). Diastolic dysfunction predicts new-onset atrial fibrillation and cardiovascular events in patients with acute myocardial infarction and depressed left ventricular systolic function: a CARISMA substudy. *Eur J Echocardiogr* 11: 602–7.

Jover E, Marin F, Roldan V, Montoro-Garcia S, Valdes M, Lip G (2013). Atherosclerosis and thromboembolic risk in atrial fibrillation: focus on peripheral vascular disease. *Ann Med* 45: 274–300.

Junttila MJ, Gonzalez M, Lizotte E, Benito B, Vernooy K, Sarkozy A, et al. (2008). Induced Brugada-type electrocardiogram, a sign for imminent malignant arrhythmias. *Circulation* 8: 1890–3.

Kaab S, Darbar D, van Noord C, et al. (2009). Large scare replication and meta-analysis of variants on chromosome 4q25 associated with atrial fibrillation. *Eur Heart J* 30: 813–19.

Karasoy D, Jensen TB, Hansen ML, Schmiegelow M, Lamberts M, Gislason GH, et al. (2013). Obesity is a risk factor for atrial fibrillation among fertile young women: a nationwide cohort study. *Europace* 15: 781–6.

Kato T, Yamashita T, Sagara K, Iinuma H, Fu LT (2004). Progressive nature of paroxysmal atrial fibrillation: observations from a 14-year follow-up study. *Circ J* 68: 568–72.

Kaw R, Hernandez AV, Masood I, Gillinov AM, Saliba W, Blackstone EH (2011). Short- and long-term mortality associated with new-onset atrial fibrillation after coronary artery bypass grafting: a systematic review and meta-analysis. *J Thorac Cardiovasc Surg* 141: 1305–12.

Kerr CR, Humphries KH, Talajic M, Klein GJ, Connolly SJ, Green M, et al. (2005). Progression to chronic atrial fibrillation after the initial diagnosis of paroxysmal atrial fibrillation: results from the Canadian Registry of Atrial Fibrillation. *American Heart J* 3: 489–96.

Kim MH, Johnston SS, Chu B, Dalal MR, Schulman KL (2011). Estimation of total incremental health care costs in patients with atrial fibrillation in the United States. *Circ Cardiovasc Quad Outcomes* 4: 313–20.

Kodama S, Saito K, Tanaka S, Horikawa C, Saito A, Heianza Y, et al. (2011). Alcohol consumption and risk of atrial fibrillation. *J Am Coll Cardiol* 57: 427–36.

Krijthe BP, Kunst A, Benjamin EJ, Lip GYH, Franco OH, Hofman A, et al. (2013). Projections on the number of individuals with atrial fibrillation in the European Union, from 2000-2006. *Eur Heart J* 34(55): 2746–51.

Krishnamoorthy S, Lip GYH, Lane DA (2009). Alcohol and illicit drug use as precipitants of atrial fibrillation in young adults: a case series and literature review. *The American Journal of Medicine* 122: 851–6.

Kubo T, Kitaoka H, Okawa M, Hirota T, Hayato K, Yamazaki N, et al. (2009). Clinical impact of atrial fibrillation in patients with hypertrophic cardiomyopathy: results from Kochi RYOMA study. *Circ J* 73: 1599–605.

Kusano KF, Taniyama M, Nakamura K, Miura D, Banba K, Nagase S, et al. (2008). Atrial fibrillation in patients with Brugada syndrome relationships of gene mutation, electrophysiology, and clinical backgrounds. *J Am Coll Cardiol* 25: 1169–75.

Lenihan CR, Montez-Rath ME, Scandling JD, Turakhia MP, Winkelmayer WC (2013). Outcomes after kidney transplantation of patients previously diagnosed with atrial fibrillation. *Am J Transplant* 13: 1566–75.

Lappegard KT, Hovland A, Pop GAM, Mollnes TE (2013). Atrial fibrillation: inflammation in disguise? *Scand J Immunol* 78: 112–19.

Li J, Solus J, Chen Q, Rho YH, Milne G, Stein M, et al. (2010). Role of inflammation and oxidative stress in atrial fibrillation. *Heart Rhythm* 7: 438–44.

Link MS, Luttmann-Gibson H, Schwartz J, Mittleman MA, Wessler B, Gold Dr, et al. (2013). Acute exposure to air pollution triggers atrial fibrillation. *J Am Coll Cardiol* 62: 816–25.

Lloyd-Jones D, Adams RJ, Brown TM, Carnethon M, Dai S, Simone GD, et al. (2010). Heart disease and stroke statistics- 2010 update: a report from the American Heart Association. *Circulation* 121: e46–215.

Lloyd-Jones DM, Wang TJ, Leip EP, Larson MG, Levy D, Vasan RS, et al. (2004). Lifetime risk for development of atrial fibrillation: the Framingham Heart Study. *Circulation* 110: 1042–6.

Loke YK, Jeevanantham V, Singh S (2009). Bisphosphonates and atrial fibrillation systematic review and meta-analysis. *Drug Saf* 32(3): 219–28.

Lubitz SA, Benjamin EJ, Ruskin JN, Fuster V, Ellinor PT (2010a). Challenges in the classification of atrial fibrillation. *Nat Rev Cardiol* 7(8): 451–60.

Lubitz SA, Moser C, Sullivan L, Rienstra M, Fontes JD, Villalon ML, et al. (2013). Atrial fibrillation patterns and risks of subsequent stroke, heart failure, or death in the community. *J Am Heart Assoc* 2: e000126.

Lubitz SA, Ozcan C, Magnani JW, Kaab S, Benjamin EJ, Ellinor PT (2010b). Genetics of atrial fibrillation: implications for future research directions and personalized medicine. *Circ Arrhythm Electrophysiol* 3: 291–9.

Lubitz SA, Rienstra M (2013). Genetic susceptibility to atrial fibrillation: does heart failure change our perspective? *Eur J Heart Fail* 15: 244–6.

Lubitz SA, Rosen AB, Ellinor PT, Benjamin EJ (2010c). Stroke risk in AF: do AF patterns matter? *Eur Heart J* 31: 908–10.

Lubitz SA, Yin X, Fontes JD, Magnani JW, Rienstra M, Pai M, et al. (2010d). Association between familial atrial fibrillation and risk of new-onset atrial fibrillation. *JAMA* 304(20): 2263–9.

Magnani JW, Hylek EM, Apovian CM (2013). Obesity begets atrial fibrillation: a contemporary summary. *Circulation* 128: 401–5.

Magnani JW, Moser CB, Murabito JM, Nelson KP, Fontes JD, Lubitz SA, et al. (2012). Age of natural menopause and atrial fibrillation: the Framingham Heart Study. *Am Heart J* 163: 729–34.

Magnani JW, Rienstra M, Lin H, Sinner MF, Lubitz SA, McManus DD, et al. (2011). Atrial fibrillation current knowledge and future directions in epidemiology and genomics. *Circulation* 124: 1982–93.

Maisel WH, Stevenson LW (2003). Atrial fibrillation in heart failure: epidemiology, pathophysiology, and rationale for therapy. *Am J Cardiol* 91: 2D–8D.

Manolis AJ, Rosel EA, Coca A, Cifkova R, Erdine, SE, Kjeldsen S, et al. (2012). Hypertension and atrial fibrillation: diagnostic approach, prevention and treatment. *J Hypertens* 30: 239–52.

Marinigh R, Lane DA, Lip GYH (2011). Severe renal impairment and stroke prevention in atrial fibrillation. *J Am Coll Cardiol*. 57: 1339–48.

Mariscalco G, Klersy C, Zanobini M, Banach M, Ferrarese S, Borsani P, et al. (2008). Atrial fibrillation after isolated coronary surgery affects late survival. *Circulation* 118: 1612–18.

Maron BJ, Olivotto I, Bellone P, Conte MR, Cecchi F, Flygenring BP, et al. (2002). Clinical profile of stroke in 900 patients with hypertrophic cardiomyopathy. *J Am Coll Cardiol* 39: 301–7.

Matthew JP, Fontes ML, Tudor IC, Ramsay J, Duke P, Mazer CD, et al. (2004). A multicenter risk index for atrial fibrillation after cardiac surgery. *JAMA* 291: 1720–9.

McClaskey D, Lee D, Buch E (2013). Outcomes among athletes and arrhythmias and electrocardiographic abnormalities: implications for ECG interpretations. *Sports Med* 43: 979–91.

McManus DD, Hsu G, Sung SH, Saczynski JS, Smith DH, Madig DJ, et al. (2013). Atrial fibrillation and outcomes in heart failure with preserved versus reduced left ventricular ejection fraction. *J Am Heart Assoc* 2(e005694): 1–9.

Mehall JR, Kohut RM Jr, Schneeberger EW, Merrill WH, Wolf RK (2007). Absence of correlation between symptoms and rhythm in "symptomatic" atrial fibrillation. *Ann Thorac Surg* 83(6): 2118–21.

Melacini P, Basso C, Angelini A, Calore C, Bobbo F, Tokajuk B, et al. (2010). Clinicopathilogical profiles of progressive heart failure in hypertrophic cardiomyopathy. *Eur Heart J* 31: 2111–23.

Menezes AR, Lavie CJ, DiNicolantonio JJ, O'Keefe J, Morin DP, Khatib S, et al. (2013). Atrial fibrillation in the 21st century: a current understand of risk factors and primary prevention strategies. *Mayo Clin Proc* 88: 394–409.

Mitchell GF, Vasan RS, Keyes MJ, Parise H, Wang TJ, Larson MG, et al. (2007). Pulse pressure and risk of new-onset atrial fibrillation. *JAMA* 297(7): 709–15.

Mittal S, Movsowski C, Steinberg JS (2011). Ambulatory external electrocardiographic monitoring: focus on atrial fibrillation. *J Am Coll Cardiol* 58: 1741–9.

Miyasaka Y, Barnes ME, Bailey KR, Cha SS, Gersh BJ, Seward JB, et al. (2007). Mortality trends in patients diagnosed with first atrial fibrillation: a 21-year community study. *J Am Coll Cardiol* 49: 986–92.

Miyasaka Y, Barnes ME, Gersh BJ, Cha SS, Bailey KR, Abhayaratna W, *et al.* (2006). Incidence and mortality risk of congestive heart failure in atrial fibrillation patients: a community-based study over two decades. *Eur Heart J* 27: 936–41.

Morrison TB, Bunch TJ, Gersh BJ (2009). Pathophysiology of concomitant atrial fibrillation and heart failure: implications for management. *Nat Clin Pract Cardiovasc Med* 6: 46–56.

Monahan K, Storfer-Isser A, Mehra R, Shahar E, Mittleman M, Rottman J, *et al.* (2009). Triggering of nocturnal arrhythmias by sleep disordered breathing events. *J Am Coll Cardiol* 54(9): 1797–804.

Mountantonakis SE, Grau-Sepulveda MV, Bhatt DL, Hernandez AF, Peterson ED, Fonarow GC (2012). Presence of atrial fibrillation is independently associated with adverse outcomes in patients hospitalized with heart failure: an analysis of get with the guidelines—heart failure. *Circ Heart Fail* 5: 191–201.

Mukamal K, Tolstrup J, Friberg J, Jensen G, Gronbaek M (2005). Alcohol consumption and risk of atrial fibrillation in men and women: the Copenhagen City Heart Study. *Circulation* 112: 1736–42.

Nattel S, Harada M (2014). Atrial remodeling and atrial fibrillation: recent advances and translational perspectives. *JACC* 63: 2335–45.

Nattel S, Maguy A, Le Bouter S, Yeh YH (2007). Arrhythmogenic ion-channel remodeling in the heart: heart failure, myocardial infarction, and atrial fibrillation. *Physiol Rev* 87: 425–56.

Nichols GA, Reinier K, Chugh SS (2009). Independent contribution of diabetes to increased prevalence and incidence of atrial fibrillation. *Diabetes Care* 32: 1851–6.

Nielsen JB, Graff C, Pietersen A, Lind B, Struijk JJ, Olesen MS, *et al.* (2013). J-shaped association between qtc interval duration and the risk of atrial fibrillation. *J Am Coll Cardiol* 61: 2557–64.

Nieuwlaat R, Capucci A, Camm AJ, Olsson SB, Andersen D, Davies DW, *et al.* (2005). Atrial fibrillation management: a prospective survey in ESC member countries: the Euro Heart Survey on Atrial Fibrillation. *Eur Heart J* 26: 2422–34.

Nieuwlaat R, Prins MH, Le Heuzey JY, Vardas PE, Aliot E, Santini M, *et al.* (2008). Prognosis, disease progression, and treatment of atrial fibrillation patients during 1 year: follow-up of the Euro Heart Survey on atrial fibrillation. *Eur Heart J* 29: 1181–9.

Nimmo C, Wright M, Goldsmith D (2013). Management of atrial fibrillation in chronic kidney disease: double trouble. *Am Heart J* 166: 230–9.

Ohe T (2009). Results from the Kochi RYOMA study: atrial fibrillation is a major risk of morbidity in patients with hypertrophic cardiomyopathy. *Circ J* 73: 1589–90.

O'Keefe JH, Bhatti SK, Patil HR, DiNicolantonio JJ, Lucan SC, Lavie CJ (2013). Effects of habitual coffee consumption on cardiometabolic disease, cardiovascular health, and all-cause mortality. *J Am Coll Cardiol* 62: 1043–51.

Okin PM, Bang CN, Wachtell K, Hille DA, Kjeldsen SE, Dahlof B, *et al.* (2013). Relationship of sudden cardiac death to new-onset atrial fibrillation in hypertensive patients with left ventricular hypertrophy. *Circ Arrhythm Electrophysiol* 6: 243–51.

Okin PM, Wachtell K, Devereux RB, Harris KE, Jern S, Kjeldsen SE, *et al.* (2006). Regression of electrocardiographic left ventricular hypertrophy and decreased incidence of new-onset atrial fibrillation: the LIFE study. *JAMA* 296: 1242–8.

Olesen JB, Lip GYH, Kamper A, Hommel K, Kober L, Lane DA, *et al.* (2012). Stroke and bleeding in atrial fibrillation with chronic kidney disease. *N Engl J Med* 367: 625–35.

Olesen JB, Lip GYH, Lane DA (2011). An epidemic of atrial fibrillation? *Europace* 13: 1059–60.

Olivotto I, Cecchi F, Casey SA, Dolara A, Traverse JH, Maron BJ, *et al.* (2001). Impact of atrial fibrillation on the clinical course of hypertrophic cardiomyopathy. *Circulation* 104: 2517–24.

Olshansky B (2005). Interrelationships between the autonomic nervous system and atrial fibrillation. *Prog Cardiovasc Dis* 48(1): 57–78.

Olsson LG, Swedberg K, Ducharme A, Granger CB, Michelson EL, McMurray JJV, *et al.* (2006). Atrial fibrillation and risk of clinical events in chronic heart failure with and without left ventricular systolic dysfunction. *J Am Coll Cardiol* 47: 1997–2004.

Omae T, Kanmura Y (2012). Management of postoperative atrial fibrillation. *J Anesth* 26(3): 429–37.

Page RL (2004). Clinical practice. Newly diagnosed atrial fibrillation. *N Engl J Med* 55: 700–7.

Pappone C, Radinovic A, Manguso F, Vicedomini G, Ciconte G, Sacchi S, *et al.* (2008). Atrial fibrillation progression and management: a 5-year prospective follow-up study. *Heart Rhythm* 5: 1501–7.

Patel D, Mohanty P, Di Biase L, Shaheen M, Lewis WR, Quan K, *et al.* (2010). Safety and efficacy of pulmonary vein antral isolation in patients with obstructive sleep apnea. *Circ Arrhythm Electrophysiol* 3: 445–51

Pedersen OD, Abildstrom SZ, Ottesen MM, Rask-Madsen C, Bagger H, Kober L, *et al.* (2006). Increased risk of sudden and non-sudden cardiovascular death in patients with atrial fibrillation/flutter following myocardial infarction. *Eur Heart J* 27: 290–5.

Perez MV, Wang PJ, Larson JC, Soliman EZ, Limacher M, Rodriguez B, *et al.* (2013). Risk factors for atrial fibrillation and their population burden in postmenopausal women: the Women's Health Initiative Observational Study. *Heart* 99: 1173–8.

Piccini JP, Stevens SR, Chang Y, Singer DE, Lokhnygina Y, Go AS, *et al.* (2013). Renal dysfunction as a predictor of stroke and systemic embolism in patients with nonvalvular atrial fibrillation: validation of the R2CHADS2 index in the ROCKET AF (Rivaroxaban vitamin K antagonism for prevention of stroke and embolism trial in atrial fibrillation) and the ATRIA (AnTicoagulation and risk factors in atrial fibrillation) study cohorts. *Circulation* 127: 224–32.

Pizzale S, Gollob MH, Gow R, Birnie DH (2008). Sudden death in a young man with catecholaminergic polymorphic ventricular tachycardia and paroxysmal atrial fibrillation. *J Cardiovasc Electrophysiol* 19: 1319–21.

Postema PG, Wolpert C, Amin AS, Probst V, Borggrefe M, Roden DM, *et al.* (2009). Drugs and Brugada syndrome patients: review of the literature, recommendations, and an up-to-date website. *Heart Rhythm* 6: 1335–41.

Potpara TS, Polovina MM, Licina MM, Marinkovic JM, Prostran MS, Lip GYH (2012). Reliable identification of "truly low" thromboembolic risk in patients initially diagnosed with "lone" atrial fibrillation: The Belgrade Atrial Fibrillation Study. *Circ Arrhythm Electrophysiol* 5: 319–26.

Prystowsky EN (2008). The history of atrial fibrillation: the last 100 years. *J Cardiovasc Electrophysiol* 19(6): 575–82.

Rader F, Van Wagoner DR, Ellinor PT, Gillinov AM, Chung MK, Costantini O, *et al.* (2011). Influence of race on atrial fibrillation after cardiac surgery. *Circulation* 4: 644–52.

Raman SV (2010). The hypertensive heart: an integrated understanding informed by imaging. *J Am Coll Cardiol* 55: 91–6.

Rho RW (2009). The management of atrial fibrillation after cardiac surgery. *Heart* 95: 422–9.

Rienstra M, Lubitz SA, Mahida S, Magnani JW, Fontes JD, Sinner MF, *et al.* (2012a). Symptoms and functional status of patients with atrial fibrillation: state of the art and future research opportunities. *Circulation* 125: 2933–43.

Rienstra M, McManus DD, Benjamin EJ (2012b). Novel risk factors for atrial fibrillation, useful for risk prediction and clinical decision making? *Circulation.* 125: e941–6.

Rivero-Ayerza M, op Reimer WS, Lenzen M, Theuns DAMJ, Jordaens L, Komajda M, *et al.* (2008). New-onset atrial fibrillation is an independent predictor of in-hospital mortality in hospitalized heart failure patients: results of the EuroHeart Failure Survey. *Eur Heart J* 29: 1618–24.

Rodríguez-Mañero M, Namdar M, Sarkozy A, Casado-Arroyo R, Ricciardi D, de Asmundis C, *et al.* (2013). Prevalence, clinical characteristics and management of atrial fibrillation in patients with Brugada syndrome. *Am J Cardiol* 111: 362–7.

Roger VL, Go AS, Lloyed-Jones DM, *et al.* (2012). Heart disease and stroke statistics-2012 update: a report from the American Heart Associate. *Circulation* 125(1): e2–220.

Rosenberg MA, Manning WJ (2012). Diastolic dysfunction and risk of atrial fibrillation: a mechanistic appraisal. *Circulation* 126: 2353–62.

Rosso R, Sparks PB, Morton JB, Kistler PM, Vohra JK, Halloran K, *et al.* (2010). Vagal paroxysmal atrial fibrillation: prevalence and ablation outcome in patients without structural heart disease. *J Cardiovasc Electrophysiol* 21: 489–93.

Roy D, Talajic M, Dubuc M, Thibault B, Guerra P, Laurent M, *et al.* (2009). Atrial fibrillation and congestive heart failure. *Cur Opin Cardiol* 24: 29–34.

Sanna T, Diener HC, Passman RS, Di Lazzaro V, Bernstein RA, Morillo CA, *et al.* (2014). Cryptogenic Stroke and Underlying Atrial Fibrillation. *N Engl J Med* 370: 2478–2486.

Savelieva I, Camm J (2004). Atrial Fibrillation and heart failure: natural history and pharmacological treatment. *Europace* 5: S5–19.

Schnabel RB, Larson MG, Yamamoto JF, Sullivan LM, Pencina MJ, Meigs JB, et al. (2010). Relations of biomarkers of distinct pathophysiological pathways and atrial fibrillation incidence in the community. *Circulation* 121: 200–7.

Schnabel RB, Sullivan LM, Levy D, Pencina MJ, Massaro JM, D'Acostino Sr RB, et al. (2009). Development of a risk score for atrial fibrillation (Framingham Heart Study): a community-based cohort study. *Lancet* 373: 739–45.

Seet R, Friedman PA, Rabinstein AA (2011). Prolonged rhythm monitoring for the detection of occult paroxysmal atrial fibrillation in ischemic stroke of unknown cause. *Circulation* 124: 477–86.

Selmer C, Olesen JB, Hansen ML, Lindhardsen J, Olsen AS, Madsen JC, et al. (2012). The spectrum of thyroid disease and risk of new onset atrial fibrillation: a large population cohort study. *BMJ* 345: e7895.

Schoonderwoerd BA, Smit MD, Pen L, Van Gelder IC (2008). New risk factors for atrial fibrillation: causes of 'not-so-lone atrial fibrillation.' *Europace* 10: 668–73.

Shenasa M, Soleimanieh M, Shenasa F (2012). Individualized therapy in patients with atrial fibrillation: new look at atrial fibrillation. *Europace* 14: v121–4.

Smith JG, Melander O, Sjogren M, Hedblad B, Engstrom G, Newton-Cheh C, et al. (2013). Genetic polymorphisms confer risk of atrial fibrillation in patients with heart failure: a population based study. *Eur J Heart Fail* 15(3): 250–7.

Sun Y, Hu D (2010). The link between diabetes and atrial fibrillation: cause or correlation. *J Cardiovasc Dis Res* 1(1): 10–11.

Tang RB, Dong JZ, Liu XP (2009). Obstructive sleep apnoea risk profile and the risk of recurrence of atrial fibrillation after catheter ablation. *Europace*. 11: 100–5.

Tedrow UB, Conen D, Ridker PM, Cook NR, Koplan BA, Manson JE, et al. (2010). The long-and short-term impact of elevated body mass index on the risk of new atrial fibrillation: The WHS (Women's Health Study). *J Am Coll Cardiol* 55: 2319–27.

The SPAF III Writing Committee for the Stroke Prevention in Atrial Fibrillation Investigators (1998). Patients with nonvalvular atrial fibrillation at low risk of stroke during treatment with aspirin: Stroke Prevention in Atrial Fibrillation Study. *JAMA* 279: 1273–7.

Tsang TSM, Barnes ME, Miyasaka Y, Cha SS, Bailey KR, Verzosa GC, et al. (2008). Obesity as a risk factor for the progression of paroxysmal to permanent atrial fibrillation: a longitudinal cohort study of 21 years. *Eur Heart J* 29: 2227–33.

Tsang TSM, Gersh BJ, Appleton CP, Tajik AJ, Barnes ME, Bailey KR, et al. (2002). Left ventricular diastolic dysfunction as a predictor of the first diagnosed nonvalvular atrial fibrillation in 840 elderly men and women. *J Am Coll Cardiol* 40: 1636–44.

Velagapudi P, Turagam MK, Leal MA, Kocheril AG (2013). Atrial fibrosis: a risk stratifier for atrial fibrillation. *Expert Rev Cardiovasc Ther* 11(2): 155–60.

Verdecchia P, Reboldi R, Bentivoglio M, Borgioni C, Angeli F, Carluccio E, et al. (2003). Atrial fibrillation in hypertension: predictors and outcome. *Hypertension* 41: 218–23.

Verma A, Champagne J, Sapp J, Essebag V, Novak P, Skanes A, et al. (2013). Discerning the incidence of symptomatic and asymptomatic episodes of atrial fibrillation before and after catheter ablation (DISCERN AF). *Arch Intern Med* 173(2): 149–56.

Vermeer SE, Prins ND, Heijer T, Hofman A, Koudstall PJ, Breteler MMB (2003). Silent brain infarcts and the risk of dementia and cognitive decline. *N Engl J Med* 348: 1215–22.

Wachter R, Stahrenberg R, Groschel K (2013). Subclinical atrial fibrillation: how hard should we look? *Heart* 99(3): 151–3.

Wakili R, Voigt N, Kääb S, Dobrev D, Nattel S (2011). Recent advances in the molecular pathophysiology of atrial fibrillation. *J Clin Invest* 121(8): 2955–68.

Waldo AL (2013). More musing about the inter-relationships of atrial fibrillation and atrial flutter and their clinical implications. *Circulation* 6: 453–4.

Wang TJ (2011). Assessing the role of circulating, genetic, and imaging biomarkers in cardiovascular risk prediction. *Circulation* 123: 551–65.

Wang TJ, Larson MG, Levy D, Vasan RS, Leip EP, Wolf PA, et al. (2003). Temporal relations of atrial fibrillation and their joint influence on mortality: the Framingham Heart Study. *Circulation* 107: 2920–5.

Wang TJ, Parise H, Levy D, D'Agostino RB, Wolf PA, Vasan RS, et al. (2004). Obesity and the risk of new-onset atrial fibrillation. *JAMA* 292: 2471–7.

Watanabe H, Watanabe T, Sasaki S, Nagai K, Roden DM, Aizawa Y (2009). Close bidirectional relationship between chronic kidney disease and atrial fibrillation: the Niigata preventive medicine study. *Am Heart J* 158: 629–36.

Wilkinson GS, Baillargeon J, Kuo YF, Freeman JL, Goodwin JS (2010). Atrial fibrillation and stroke associated with intravenous bisphosphate therapy in older patients with cancer. *J Clin Oncol* 28: 4898–905.

Winkelmayer WC (2013). More evidence on an abominable pairing: atrial fibrillation and kidney disease. *Circulation* 127: 560–2.

Wongcharoen W, Chen SA (2012). The pathophysiology of atrial fibrillation in heart failure. *J Innovat Cardiac Rhythm Manag* 3: 865–9.

Wyse GD, Van Gelder IC, Ellinor PT, Go AS, Kalman JM, Narayan SM, *et al.* (2014). Lone atrial fibrillation: does it exist? *JACC* 63(17): 1715–23.

Zakeri R, Chamberlain AM, Roger VL, Redfield MM (2013). Temporal relationship and prognostic significance of atrial fibrillation in heart failure patients with preserved ejection fraction: a community-based study. *Circulation* 128: 1085–93.

Zhuang J, Yuyan L, Tang K, Peng W, Xu Y (2013). Influence of body mass index on recurrence and quality of life in atrial fibrillation patients after catheter ablation: a meta-analysis and systematic review. *Clin Cardiol* 36(5): 269–75.

Zimetbaum P, Goldman A (2010). Ambulatory arrhythmia monitoring: choosing the right device. *Circulation* 122: 1629–36.

Zöller B, Ohlsson H, Sundquist J, Sundquist K (2012). High familial risk of atrial fibrillation/atrial flutter in multiplex families: a nationwide family study in Sweden. *J Am Heart Assoc* 1(e003384): 1–9.

Chapter 5

Use of antiarrhythmic drug treatment in atrial fibrillation

Irene Savelieva and A. John Camm

> **Key points**
>
> - Despite several trials demonstrating non-inferiority of rate control to rhythm control, with some advantages to the former, rhythm control is the preferred treatment strategy in young and active individuals and those who remain symptomatic despite best possible rate control; nevertheless, rate control is relevant to all forms of AF and to all patients with AF.
>
> - The choice of an antiarrhythmic drug should be driven by its safety (preferably the effect on hard endpoints such as mortality if available) which, in turn, is determined by the underlying cardiovascular disease and other individual patient characteristics (e.g. co-morbidities and concomitant medication).
>
> - Dronedarone can be used safely in patients with non-permanent atrial fibrillation provided they do not have unstable or advanced heart failure; the drug is better avoided or should be used with caution in individuals with milder forms of heart failure unless there is no alternative
>
> - Regular electrocardiogram monitoring as well as biochemistry and functional tests (specific for each drug) are mandatory.
>
> - In selected patients, short-term use of antiarrhythmic drugs after cardioversion or a 'pill-in-the-pocket' strategy can be used in order to minimize the adverse effects.

5.1 Principles of therapy

The main principles of atrial fibrillation (AF) management consist of risk assessment for stroke and appropriate antithrombotic prophylaxis, usually in the form of oral anticoagulation; rhythm control therapy aimed at prevention of recurrent paroxysmal or persistent AF which may include antiarrhythmic drugs, catheter ablation, and cardioversion of arrhythmia which fails to self-terminate; control of ventricular rates during recurrent or permanent AF; and treatment of the conditions that are commonly associated with the occurrence and perpetuation of AF (Camm et al. 2010). The nature of AF and of individual patient factors change over time, requiring a flexible approach to long-term management. Treatment of underlying heart disease (e.g. stringent blood pressure control in hypertension) may *per se* deter the occurrence of AF by prevention of atrial remodelling and is likely to contribute to the reduction of recurrence and delay progression to permanent AF.

AF often occurs without causing any symptoms and is discovered by the finding of an irregular pulse or an abnormal electrocardiogram (ECG) (Savelieva and Camm 2000). This

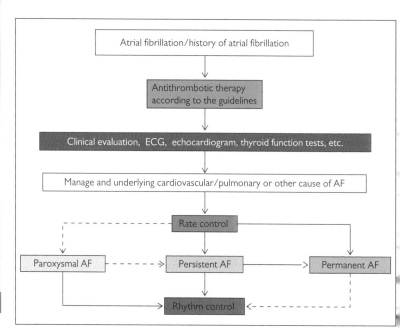

Figure 5.1 Algorithm outlining the management of newly diagnosed AF and the process of choosing between rhythm and rate control strategies on the basis of AF subtype. Solid lines: initial approach; dashed lines: secondary approach; dotted lines last resort.

patient needs urgent assessment of thromboembolic risk and, if appropriate and as far as possible, prompt evaluation and correction of underlying cardiovascular disease (Figure 5.1). The heart rate during AF should be evaluated by ECG, exercise testing, or 24-hour ambulatory ECG monitoring. If necessary, rate control therapy should be instituted. If the patient remains asymptomatic, nothing further needs to be done, unless there is evidence to believe that the AF is of recent onset or is non-permanent in nature. It is then appropriate to consider whether a rhythm control approach might be attempted, on the basis that if sinus rhythm is restored the patient might feel much better than when in AF. It also should be recognized that older patients with non-specific symptoms such as exertional shortness of breath, reduced exercise tolerance, and fatigue often blame their symptoms on 'old age' and accommodate to the symptoms by lowering their expectations, and adjusting their lifestyle to limitations imposed by the disease.

5.1.1. **Progression of atrial fibrillation**

Furthermore, deterring the rhythm control treatment may impede success of restoration and/or maintenance of sinus rhythm in the future. In the RECORD-AF (REgistry on Cardiac rhythm disORDers assessing control of Atrial Fibrillation) registry, if rate control was selected as the initial treatment strategy for new-onset paroxysmal AF, the likelihood of progression to persistent or permanent AF over the subsequent year was threefold higher than with rhythm control (Figure 5.2) (De Vos et al. 2012). Generally, progression from paroxysmal AF to persistent or permanent AF occurs at the rate of

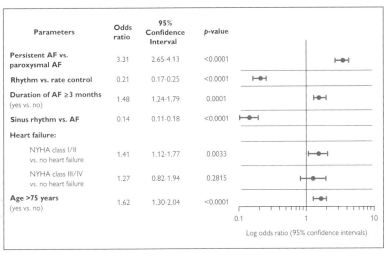

Parameters	Odds ratio	95% Confidence Interval	p-value
Persistent AF vs. paroxysmal AF	3.31	2.65-4.13	<0.0001
Rhythm vs. rate control	0.21	0.17-0.25	<0.0001
Duration of AF ≥3 months (yes vs. no)	1.48	1.24-1.79	0.0001
Sinus rhythm vs. AF	0.14	0.11-0.18	<0.0001
Heart failure:			
NYHA class I/II vs. no heart failure	1.41	1.12-1.77	0.0033
NYHA class III/IV vs. no heart failure	1.27	0.82-1.94	0.2815
Age >75 years (yes vs. no)	1.62	1.30-2.04	<0.0001

Log odds ratio (95% confidence intervals)

Figure 5.2 Multivariate analysis of baseline factors predicting progression to permanent in the RecordAF registry. NYHA = New York Heart Association. Reproduced from *Journal of the American College of Cardiology*, A. John Camm *et al.*, Real-Life Observations of Clinical Outcomes With Rhythm- and Rate-Control Therapies for Atrial Fibrillation: RECORDAF (Registry on Cardiac Rhythm Disorders Assessing the Control of Atrial Fibrillation), 58:5, Copyright 2011 with permission from Elsevier.

5–15% per year and also depends on age at presentation and the presence of underlying heart disease (Kerr et al. 2005; De Vos et al. 2012). Patients with lone AF have the lowest progression rates of around 1–2% per year, with a small proportion remaining stable over decades (Jahangir et al. 2007). Progression of AF relates to progression of the underlying disease and to continuous structural remodelling of the atria, including changes associated with ageing (e.g. fatty metamorphosis, myocyte degeneration, and fibrosis). As the arrhythmia becomes more sustained, restoration and maintenance of sinus rhythm become more challenging and some, therefore, advocate early aggressive rhythm control (Cosio et al. 2008).

When the patient presents with symptoms of AF (e.g. palpitations, anxiety, breathlessness, or chest pain), heart rate should be slowed, usually by using an intravenous beta blocker or rate-limiting calcium channel blocker. If the patient remains symptomatic, or is haemodynamically compromised, early cardioversion with appropriate thromboembolic protection (see Chapter 6) is justified. Otherwise a decision must be made, on a case-by-case basis, of the merits of adopting a rate or rhythm control management strategy. Although randomized controlled trials have usually concluded that there is little to choose between these strategies with regard to major cardiovascular outcomes (Van Gelder et al. 2002; Wyse et al. 2002; Roy et al. 2008) (Figure 5.3), most physicians tend to choose a rhythm control strategy in those who are young, active, or symptomatic especially if there is little underlying cardiovascular disease (good left ventricular function and near normal left atrial size). On the other hand, in older, sedentary, asymptomatic patients with significant heart disease a rate control strategy often proves easier and more reliable.

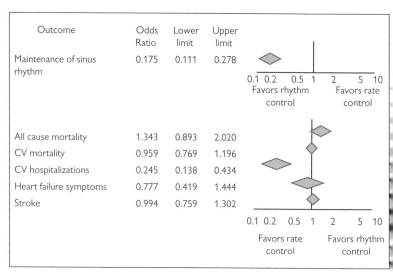

Figure 5.3 Composite of the results of meta-analyses of rate versus rhythm control.
CV = cardiovascular. Source data from Al-Khatib SM, et al. AHRQ Publication No.13-EHC095-EF.
Rockville, MD: Agency for Healthcare Research and Quality; June 2013.

5.2 **Rate control**

This may be applied as an initial therapy for all forms of AF, and is the definitive treatment for AF which is considered to be permanent in nature. Very rapid ventricular rates cause palpitations and other rate-related symptoms, but rates which are faster than normal, but insufficient to be directly symptomatic, may lead to degradation of left ventricular performance, mitral regurgitation, and left atrial dilation. This may be very obvious with persistent heart rates more than 125 beats per minute (bpm) when even a normal ventricle may dilate, but in patients with existing poor ventricular function less high resting rates, for example, above 100 bpm may aggravate left ventricular dysfunction and precipitate heart failure. On the other hand, loss of atrial contraction which typically provides approximately 20–30% of the total stroke volume, may lead to a significant reduction in cardiac output, especially in patients with impaired diastolic filling, hypertensive heart disease, and left ventricular hypertrophy. Ventricular irregularity also contributes to reduced cardiac output. For these reasons, it has been assumed that the heart rate during AF should be controlled to be at or slightly above the physiological range, for example, below 80 bpm at rest and 110 bpm on moderate exercise (Van Gelder et al. 2006).

Recent data suggest that asymptomatic patients may be sufficiently well controlled if the rate at rest is below 100–110 bpm. The RACE (RAte Control Efficacy) II study in 614 patients with permanent AF has found no significant difference in clinically relevant outcomes such as cardiovascular mortality, hospitalization for heart failure, stroke, major bleeding, ventricular tachyarrhythmias, etc., between lenient (resting heart rate < 110 bpm) and strict (resting heart rate < 80 bpm and heart rate during moderate exercise < 110 bpm) rate control (12.9% vs 14.9%) (Van Gelder et al. 2010). However, the study was small, follow-up was relatively short (up to 3 years), with only 75% of patients in the strict control arm achieving the target rates, and the difference between ventricular rates in two arms was not sufficient to provide definitive evidence that the degree of rate control is not important. Thus, although trial data are consistent on this point, there has not yet been a sufficiently large trial to convince physicians that it is not appropriate to be reasonably strict about achieving a resting heart rate below 80 bpm.

Furthermore, ventricular rate control at rest does not always translate into effective control during exercise. Only a limited number of studies specifically addressed the effect of rate-slowing drugs on chronotropic competence in AF or defined upper limits of the appropriate ventricular rate response during exercise (Lewis et al. 1988; Rawles 1990). Rawles (1990) demonstrated that rates of up to 90 bpm maintain good cardiac output at rest, while during exercise, ventricular rates of 90–140 bpm might be necessary in order to maintain equivalent cardiac outputs to patients in sinus rhythm.

These principles may be easy to consider in patients with permanent AF, but are more difficult to apply to patients in whom AF is intermittent (paroxysmal or persistent), because the heart rate control during the arrhythmia may not be similar to the effect on heart rate during sinus rhythm. This is especially true when sick sinus syndrome (or tachy-brady syndrome) is present. In these circumstances symptomatic bradycardia may occur and prevent adequate rate control during the arrhythmia. This may be sufficiently profound to warrant heart rate support, when not in AF, by the use of an artificial pacemaker—a dual-chamber device is essential since atrioventricular (AV) sequencing should be maintained during sinus rhythm and rapid detection of AF onset is needed when the arrhythmia occurs. Biventricular pacing may be needed if the ventricles are paced often (more than 25%). Failure to find an adequate blend of the effect on heart rate in sinus rhythm and in AF is often the main reason for the failure of rate control therapy. It should be remembered that the AV nodal effect is often more dominant with calcium channel blockers whereas sinus bradycardia is often more marked than the effect on the AV node with beta-blockers. Judicious dose adjustment with one or more of the agents may allow satisfactory rate control.

5.2.1 Drugs for ventricular rate control

Traditionally rate control may be achieved with digitalis glycosides. However, when given as a monotherapy digoxin is rarely adequate to control exercise heart rates although it may be sufficient to control resting heart rates and can therefore be useful as monotherapy in sedentary patients. Digoxin is less efficacious for rate control than rate-slowing calcium channel blockers and amiodarone, and in some studies, to beta blockers. Recently concern has been expressed about a potential increase of mortality in AF patients treated with digoxin (Whitbeck et al. 2013), and physicians are generally avoiding this therapy. Most patients should be treated with either a beta-blocker (usually a cardio-specific agent such as bisoprolol, carvedilol, metoprolol, or nebivolol) or a rate-limiting calcium channel blocker such as verapamil or diltiazem (Table 5.1) (Farshi et al. 1999; Khand et al. 2003; Olshansky et al. 2004). Beta-blockade is preferred in patents with left ventricular dysfunction and calcium channel blockers are advantageous in patients with chronic obstructive pulmonary disease. Sometimes a combination of one drug from each category is needed, although it is not advised in patients with poor ventricular function. As a last resort amiodarone is advocated, especially in patients with heart failure—it is a powerful and effective rate-limiting agent, but it has an extensive catalogue of adverse side effects.

Some antiarrhythmic drugs, such as sotalol and amiodarone, slow AV conduction and thus offer an additional benefit of ventricular rate control during recurrences of AF, but they are not commonly employed for long-term rate control because of the risk of adverse effects including proarrhythmia. This has been further reinforced by the results of the PALLAS (Permanent Atrial fibriLLAtion outcome Study using dronedarone on top

Table 5.1 Drugs for rate control in atrial fibrillation

Drug	Average mainte-nance dose	Preferable clinical setting	Potential adverse effects
Digoxin	Loading dose: 250 mcg every 2 hours; up to 1500 mcg; main-tenance dose 125–250 mcg daily	As monotherapy, used mainly in the elderly and sedentary patients; is not recommended as first-line treatment due to the limited efficacy during exercise and a potential adverse effect on survival; should be avoided in paroxysmal (and possibly, persistent) AF because of profibrillatory effects (shortens the atrial refrac-tory period)	Bradycardia; atrioventricu-lar block; atrial arrhythmias; ventricular tachycardia
Diltiazem	120–360 mg daily	First-line therapy in patients with asthma and chronic obstructive pulmonary disease	Hypotension; atrioventricu-lar block; heart failure
Verapamil	80–360 mg daily		
Atenolol	50–100 mg daily	Preferred inpatients with coronary artery disease, myocardial infarction, heart failure (specifically, bisopro-lol and carvedilol)	Hypotension; bradycardia;atrioventricullar block; deterioration of chronic obstructive pul-monary disease or asthma; fatigue
Metoprolol	50–200 mg daily		
Nebivolol	5–10 mg daily		
Bisoprolol	5–10 mg daily		
Carvedilol	25–100 mg daily		
Sotalol	80–320 mg daily	Rate-slowing effect is useful during the recurrence of atrial fibrillation; not recom-mended in permanent AF	Bradycardia; QT prolonga-tion; torsade de pointes; hypotension
Amiodarone	200 mg daily	Rate-slowing effect is useful during the recurrence of atrial fibrillation; limited use in permanent AF because of multiple toxicities; pref-erence should be given to non-pharamacological rate control ("ablate and pace")	Bradycardia; QT prolonga-tion; torsade de pointes (risk <1%); photosensitivity; pulmonary toxicity; poly-neuropathy; hepatic toxic-ity; thyroid dysfunction; gastrointestinal upset

of standard therapy) trial in which the use of dronedarone in patients with permanent AF was associated with a higher incidence of death and major adverse events compared with placebo (Connolly et al. 2011).

When rate control is impossible to achieve with AV nodal blocking drugs an interven-tional approach (AV node/His bundle ablation with pacemaker implantation) may be con-sidered (Brignole et al. 2013).

5.2.2 Assessment of rate control

The ventricular rate in AF cannot be adequately assessed by palpation of the radial pulse because close-coupled beats may not result in a mechanical response sufficiently strong to transmit to a peripheral pulse (apex–radial deficit). Apical palpation, auscultation, or preferably an ECG should be used to measure the heart rate in AF. Most patients with AF

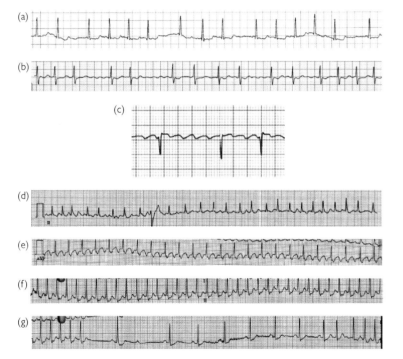

Figure 4.2 Examples of different ECG patterns of AF. (a) Fine AF. (b) Course AF. (c) Lead V₁ (same patient as (b)). (d) AF with rapid ventricular response. (e) Atrial flutter with 2:1 AV conduction. (f) AV nodal re-entrant tachycardia (same patient as (e)). (g) Termination of AVNRT to sinus rhythm with re-initiation of AF (same patient as (f)).

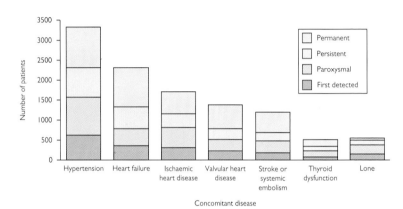

Figure 4.10 Figure illustrates types of AF according to their underlying structural heart disease. Reproduced from Nieuwlaat R, Capucci A, Camm AJ, Olsson SB, Andersen D, Davies DW, *et al*. Atrial fibrillation management: a prospective survey in ESC member countries: the Euro Heart Survey on Atrial Fibrillation. *European Heart Journal* 2005; 26: 2422–34 by permission of Oxford University Press.

are ambulant to some extent and an 'exercise' heart rate can be easily obtained from a low-level exercise testing or a 6-minute walk test (in the less fit) or 24-hour ambulatory ECG monitoring or a programmed exercise tolerance test in younger and more active patients. Twenty-four-hour ambulatory ECGs give a reliable impression of heart rate provided that patients are ambulant and not significantly exercise-limited, in which case a flat heart rate response is seen, not because of good rate control but because of limited exercise.

5.3 Rhythm control

5.3.1 What rhythm versus rate studies did not show

In the majority of rhythm versus rate control studies, a significant proportion of patients in the rhythm control arm failed to maintain sinus rhythm and many patients in the rate control arm were in sinus rhythm at the end of the study. A post hoc on-treatment analysis of the AFFIRM (Atrial Fibrillation Follow-up Investigation of Rhythm Management) trial has shown that the presence of sinus rhythm conferred a considerable reduction of 47% in mortality irrespective of the treatment strategy, but paradoxically, the use of antiarrhythmic drugs appeared to increase risk of dying (Figure 5.4) (Corley et al. 2004). However, when sinus rhythm was removed as a separate factor from the analysis, antiarrhythmic drugs were no longer associated with mortality, presumably because their beneficial effect on maintenance of sinus rhythm offset their adverse effects. In short, it suggested that in patients with AF, if sinus rhythm could be achieved safely and effectively, a favourable outcome would result. In a similar analysis from the AF-CHF (Atrial Fibrillation in Congestive Heart Failure) trial, the presence of AF (as opposed to sinus rhythm) did not predict cardiovascular or all-cause mortality once the severity of clinical symptoms and mitral regurgitation were known (Talajic et al. 2010). Unlike in the AFFIRM trial, the results of AF-CHF did

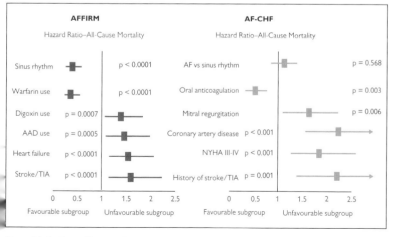

Figure 5.4 Analysis of factors influencing all-cause mortality in the AFFIRM and AF-CHF trials. AAD = antiarrhythmic drug; AF = atrial fibrillation AF-CHF = Atrial Fibrillation and Congestive Heart Failure; AFFIRM = Atrial Fibrillation Follow-up Investigation of Rhythm Management; NYHA = New York Heart Association; TIA = transient ischaemic attack.

not confirm that there was an advantage to sinus rhythm in a population of elderly patients with heart failure.

Young and symptomatic patients demanding a more aggressive approach towards restoring and maintaining sinus rhythm had been largely excluded from these studies, and the results do not apply to this AF subpopulation.

As a whole, the results of rate versus rhythm control studies highlighted the limitations of current therapies to achieve and maintain sinus rhythm. Long-term maintenance of sinus rhythm has proven difficult to achieve in patients with persistent AF, and the method is time-consuming and expensive due to the costs of the antiarrhythmic drugs and the increased need for hospitalization. The treatment of AF is beginning to change dramatically in that paroxysmal AF and some persistent AF is increasingly treated with pulmonary vein isolation and left atrial ablation prompting new rate versus rhythm control trials in younger, more active, and more symptomatic patients involving best available rhythm control therapies.

5.3.2 **Goals of antiarrhythmic drug therapy**

Rhythm control with antiarrhythmic drugs remains an essential part of AF management. The goals of prophylactic antiarrhythmic drug therapy include prevention of the recurrence of AF or modification of recurrences rendering them less symptomatic, less frequent, and less sustained or more often self-terminating. This results in the reduction of AF burden and improvement of quality of life, and also reduces the rate of progression of AF and its complications such as left ventricular dysfunction.

Antiarrhythmic drugs can be used to facilitate electrical cardioversion and to prevent early recurrence of AF. The beneficial effects include prolongation of atrial refractoriness, conversion of fibrillation to a more organized atrial rhythm (e.g. flutter) which may be cardioverted with less energy, and suppression of atrial premature beats that may re-initiate AF. Evidence for such 'synergistic' action of antiarrhythmic drugs has largely come from small studies with short-acting intravenous formulations and is limited with oral agents (Capucci et al. 2000).

In patients who underwent left atrial ablation, antiarrhythmic drugs, often at lower doses, may constitute part of 'hybrid therapy' to achieve complete suppression of the arrhythmia. It seems intuitive that effective long-term maintenance of sinus rhythm will reduce the risk of stroke, but anticoagulation should not be discontinued in patients with risk factors on the assumption that AF has been successfully suppressed.

5.3.3 **Selection of an antiarrhythmic drug**

Antiarrhythmic drugs are ion channel blockers that principally influence atrial or junctional automaticity or refractoriness in such a way to suppress the triggers of AF, such as frequent atrial premature beats, short bursts of rapid atrial tachycardia (common), or junctional reciprocating tachycardias (rare). These drugs also modulate the substrate for AF by decreasing excitability and conduction velocity, or lengthening refractoriness of atrial tissue and therefore discourage re-entry (multiple wavelets or spiral waves). Some antiarrhythmic drugs may also change the balance of autonomic stimulation of the atrial myocardium by suppression of sympathetic (e.g. beta-blockers, amiodarone, or dronedarone) or muscarinic activity (e.g. disopyramide).

The choice between antiarrhythmic drugs is usually based on side effect profiles and safety which is determined by the presence and nature of underlying heart disease rather than any specific efficacy in particular patients (Camm 2008). However, it is generally true that the most effective drugs also have the greatest propensity to cardiovascular adverse effects such as proarrhythmia (bradycardia and tachycardia) and negative inotropic effects, particularly on left ventricular function. Many patients who resort to rhythm control have already been exposed to beta-blockers for the treatment of underlying cardiovascular problems or for AF ventricular rate control, but if not, a trial of a beta-blocker is the initial approach to rhythm control, in almost every circumstance.

If optimal beta-blockade fails to be effective, is contraindicated, or is associated with adverse effects, a specific antiarrhythmic drug may be used. At this stage it is very important to consider associated cardiovascular disease. Patients are generally divided into those with no or minimal structural cardiovascular disease (lone AF), hypertensive heart disease (with or without associated significant left ventricular hypertrophy), ischaemic heart disease, or heart failure (mild or moderate to severe) (Figure 5.5). Alternatively, a classification based on left ventricular function (normal, depressed, left ventricular ejection fraction (LVEF) ≥ 35%, or < 35%) can form the primary basis for the choice of an antiarrhythmic drug.

Any of the antiarrhythmic agents can be given to patients with little or no underlying heart disease, when the choice depends on local tradition, the expense and convenience of therapy, non-cardiovascular co-morbidities or the adverse effect profile of the drug (Table 5.2). Generally amiodarone is deferred until the last resort, and sotalol is avoided because of the need for hospitalization or precautions related to the presence of AF or acquired long QT syndrome. Dofetilide and dronedarone are often kept back because of monitoring and expense issues. Generally flecainide or propafenone are the most usual first-line drugs. Patients with hypertension can be treated similarly if there is no significant left ventricular hypertrophy or likelihood of co-existing coronary heart disease.

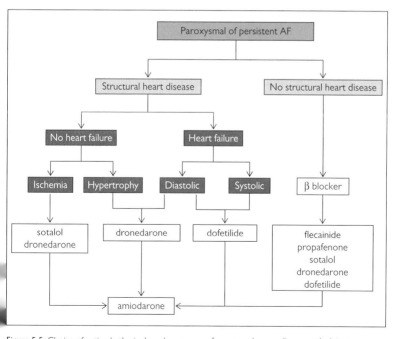

Figure 5.5 Choice of antiarrhythmic drug therapy on safety grounds according to underlying pathology.

Table 5.2 Antiarrhythmic drugs used for maintenance of sinus rhythm in patients with recurrent atrial fibrillation

Drug	Recommended dose	Average efficacy at 1 year	Main contraindications and precautions	Monitoring
Disopyramide	100–250 mg t.i.d.	54%	Contraindicated in left ventricular systolic dysfunction and in the presence of sinus node dysfunction and second- and third-degree heart block without a pacemaker Caution when using concomitant medication with QT-prolonging drugs, intraventricular conduction delay, angle-close glaucoma, prostatic enlargement	ECG: PR, QRS, QTc intervals
Flecainide	100–200 mg b.i.d.	Up to 77%	Contraindicated in coronary artery disease with evidence of myocardial ischemia, previous myocardial infarction, left ventricular systolic dysfunction Caution in the presence of conduction system disease and renal impairment	ECG: PR, QRS, QTc intervals, organization into atrial flutter Holter: atrial flutter with 1:1 or 2:1 atrioventricular conduction Renal function, particularly in the elderly patients and those with known CKD New-onset myocardial ischaemia
Flecanide XL	200 mg o.d.	Probably as above	As above	As above
Propafenone	150–300 mg t.i.d.	40–75%	Contraindicated in coronary artery disease with evidence of myocardial ischaemia, previous myocardial infarction, left ventricular systolic dysfunction Caution in the presence of conduction system disease	ECG: PR, QRS, QTc intervals, organization into atrial flutter Holter: atrial flutter with 1:1 or 2:1 atrioventricular conduction New-onset myocardial ischemia
Propafenone SR	225–425 mg b.i.d.	40–65% (dose-dependent)	As above	As above

Sotalol	80–160 mg b.i.d.	30–50%; in earlier studies up to 70%	Contraindicated in the presence of significant left ventricular hypertrophy, systolic heart failure, pre-existing QT prolongation, hypokalaemia, significant renal dysfunction Moderate renal dysfunction requires dose titration	ECG: QTc interval, heart rate Holter: ventricular tachyarrhythmias, transient repolarization abnormalities (e.g. QT prolongation, abnormal U waves) Renal function and electrolytes, particularly in the elderly patients and those with known CKD
Dofetilide	125–500 mcg b.i.d.	40–65%	Contraindicated in the presence of pre-existing QT prolongation, history or risk of torsade de pointes, creatinine clearance < 20 mL/min, hypokalaemia, hypomagnesaemia. Dose should be adjusted in accordance with creatinine clearance	ECG: QTc interval every 6 months Holter: ventricular tachyarrhythmias, transient repolarization abnormalities (e.g. QT prolongation, abnormal U waves) Renal function and electrolytes including magnesium every 6 months
Amiodarone	100–200 mg o.d.	52–70%	Caution when using concomitantly with QT prolonging drugs, heart failure Dose of warfarin and digoxin may require adjustment (reduction)	ECG: PR, QTc intervals, heart rate Holter: heart rate, transient repolarization abnormalities (e.g. QT prolongation, abnormal U waves) Creatinine. liver enzymes, thyroid hormones (every 6 months) Lung function tests (yearly), chest X-rays and/or HRCT if abnormality is detected
Dronedarone	400 mg b.i.d.	33–40%	Contraindicated in the presence of systolic heart failure NYHA class III–IV or unstable or recently decompensated heart failure, pre-existing QT prolongation, significant renal dysfunction	ECG: PR, QTc intervals, heart rate Creatinine at 7–14 days after the start of treatment and periodically thereafter Liver enzymes at 7 days after the start of treatment., monthly during the first 6 months, then at 9 and 12 months; periodically thereafter (1–2 times a year)

Some studies reported that beta blockers (bisoprolol, metoprolol, and carvedilol) were associated with a lower incidence of recurrent atrial fibrillation. However, a placebo-subtracted efficacy was modest at 12%.

Studies with Class I antiarrhythmic drugs reported an efficacy similar to that of amiodarone. However, these studies enrolled patients with no structural heart disease and with minimal left atrial remodelling who also had a relatively high rate of sinus rhythm in the placebo arm.

b.i.d. = twice daily; o.d. = once daily, t.d.s. = three times daily. CKD, chronic kidney disease; HRCT, high-resolution computed tomography.

In the presence of significant left ventricular hypertrophy, sotalol and dofetilide should be avoided because of the risk of QT prolongation and torsades de pointes, especially if potassium-wasting diuretics are also being used, for example, to manage hypertension. Conventionally flecainide and propafenone are not used because of a fear of proarrhythmia extrapolated from the results of CAST (Cardiac Arrhythmia Suppression Study) (Echt et al. 1991). Thus, only dronedarone and amiodarone are available to treat these patients and when hypertrophy is severe as in hypertrophic cardiomyopathy there has only been sufficient clinical experience to be confident about the use of amiodarone.

Flecainide and propafenone are clearly contraindicated in coronary artery disease because of increased mortality seen in the CAST study when post-myocardial infarction patients with active ischaemia were exposed to this type of drug. Sotalol, dronedarone, and amiodarone are possible treatments; each is anti-ischaemic and antiarrhythmic. Some physicians avoid sotalol and dofetilide because of the proarrhythmic risk and others prefer not to use dronedarone because of concerns related to progression to permanent AF and the burden of monitoring liver function. In the United States, dofetilide can be used but it is generally relegated until last because of the hurdles of monitoring the QT interval and potassium/magnesium levels, and the paperwork involved.

Only amiodarone and dofetilide can be considered for all grades of heart failure. In the United States, dronedarone can be used in patients with any class of heart failure and dronedarone can be given to patients with mild to moderate heart failure but not to those with recently unstable, New York Heart Association (NYHA) class IV heart failure patients, especially when LVEF is less than 35%. However, in Europe the use of dronedarone is discouraged in all patients with a history of, or current, heart failure or depressed left ventricular function. There is some concern about the use of amiodarone in NYHA class III patients, but there is little or no medical alternative in Europe. In patients with heart failure the risk of negative inotropic and proarrhythmic effects are intensified. Optimal treatment of the haemodynamic aspects of heart failure is crucial.

When there is a strong autonomic background to paroxysms of AF other consideration may apply. For example, antiarrhythmic drugs with antimuscarinic effects, such as disopyramide or quinidine, can be considered for vagotonic AF (predominantly in the setting of relative bradycardia, in the evening or at weekends, after meals, and often associated with alcohol). Drugs with strong antisympathetic actions, such as beta-blockers, dronedarone, or amiodarone, can be used for patients with paroxysms related to sympathetic stimulation (during mental or physical stress, against a background of relative sinus tachycardia).

5.3.4 **Where to initiate antiarrhythmic drug therapy?**

The site for initiation of antiarrhythmic drug therapy is determined by the underlying rhythm (AF or sinus), underlying heart disease, and other individual patient characteristics that may interfere with safety (e.g. low repolarization reserve). Patients at expectedly high risk of developing adverse effects or those in whom sinus node function is unknown and clinically significant sinus bradycardia is anticipated should be hospitalized for the initiation of antiarrhythmic drug therapy. For some antiarrhythmic agents, for example, dofetilide, there is formal requirement for in-hospital initiation.

In the absence of proarrhythmic concerns and formal labelling, convenience and cost-effectiveness favour out-of-hospital initiation. Amiodarone, dronedarone, and sotalol, due to their AV blocking effect and low risk of fast ventricular rates if AF transforms into atrial flutter, can be initiated during ongoing AF on an out-patient basis. It is also acceptable to initiate propafenone and flecainide out-of-hospital in patients with lone AF after adequate AV blockade with a beta-blocker or a rate-slowing calcium channel blocker has been ensured.

As a general rule, antiarrhythmic drugs should be started at a lower dose with upward titration, reassessing the ECG with regard to heart rate, PR and QT interval durations, QRS width, and efficacy, as each dose change is made or concomitant drug therapies are introduced. In some circumstances (e.g. long travel distance limited mobility), daily trans-telephonic monitoring can be used to provide the surveillance of the ECG parameters. Of note, even with in-hospital initiation, antiarrhythmic agents impose risk of developing proarrhythmia later in the course of therapy, which may be facilitated by progression of underlying heart disease, electrolyte abnormalities, drug interactions, and changes in absorption, metabolism, or clearance.

5.3.5 Assessment of rhythm control

It is seems straightforward to follow patients with symptomatic AF because the occurrence of symptoms suggests recurrence of the arrhythmia. However, experience with intensive ECG monitoring of patients enrolled in drug studies or following ablation procedures has demonstrated that there is often little association between symptoms and AF episodes. In many cases there are far more asymptomatic than symptomatic recurrences, and in some patients recurrences are almost always asymptomatic. Therefore it is important to consider prolonged monitoring if the recurrence of asymptomatic episodes is important to therapeutic decisions. Usually, in patients who are adequately anticoagulated silent recurrences of AF are unimportant, but if a physician intends to base decisions relating to anticoagulation or to supplementary rate control on the presence or absence of AF episodes, intensive ECG monitoring is needed, for example, 48-hour to 7-day Holter or patch monitoring ECG recording every 2 or 3 months, or even continuous monitoring with an implantable loop recorder. This form of ECG data collection is also frequently needed for research studies.

When a patient has intermittent symptoms and the likelihood of recurrence is high, but undocumented, the physician should resort to Holter ECG monitoring if the recurrences are sufficiently frequent (one or two attacks per day when 24-hour monitoring is contemplated and one or two attacks per week when 7-day ECG monitoring is proposed). Less frequent recurrences are best documented with event recorders or long-term (2–4-week) patch ECG recorders. Increasingly patients and physicians are turning to the use of smart phones with modifications to allow ECG recording and transmission to the physician or third-party vendor. When paroxysms are identified the physician should explore the mechanism of AF initiation, the stability or otherwise of the arrhythmia, and the ventricular rate during episodes of AF. Appropriate revision of treatment can then be designed.

5.4 Comparative efficacy of antiarrhythmic drugs

The superiority of one antiarrhythmic drug over another is not well documented, mainly due to a relatively small number and suboptimal design of direct comparison studies and their inconsistent results as well as enrolment of patients with different underlying cardiovascular pathologies.

5.4.1 Beta-blockers

Beta blockers are modestly effective in preventing AF (~30%) and are mainly used for rate control. An exception is adrenergically mediated AF, AF caused by thyrotoxicosis, and AF after cardiac surgery, in which case beta-blockers may be a first-line therapy. Limited evidence suggests that outside these specific settings, metoprolol was superior to placebo (Kühlkamp et al. 2000), and bisoprolol was as effective as sotalol (Plewan et al. 2001) for prevention of recurrent AF.

Some beta-blockers such as carvedilol may be more potent antiarrhythmics because of their direct effects on cardiac ion channels beyond their antiadrenergic action. In addition, carvedilol has antioxidant activity and may protect the atrial myocardium from oxidative injury caused by fast atrial rates and ischaemia. In direct comparisons, carvedilol demonstrated no benefit over bisoprolol, although a higher proportion of patients treated with carvedilol completed the 1-year study in sinus rhythm (Katritsis et al. 2003).

5.4.2 Disopyramide

Disopyramide is rarely used for treatment of AF, mainly because of its negative inotropic effect and poor tolerance due to antimuscarinic properties as well as proarrhythmias. However, the use of disopyramide is advocated in patients with lone, vagally mediated AF. In early, small studies, efficacy of disopyramide was reported to be 70% at 1 month, 67% at 6 months, and 54% at 1 year after electrical cardioversion (Karlson et al. 1988; Crijns et al. 1996). Disopyramide may be effective in patients with vagally-mediated, bradycardia-dependent AF.

5.4.3 Propafenone and flecainide

Propafenone and flecainide are recommended as first-line therapy for AF in patients without significant structural heart disease such as heart failure, hypertension with left ventricular hypertrophy, previous myocardial or coronary artery disease with documented myocardial ischaemia. Both propafenone and flecainide reduced the recurrence rate by two-thirds, with no advantage of one drug over the other. In direct comparisons, flecainide and propafenone prevented AF in 77% and 75% of patients, respectively (Chimienti et al. 1996). In a meta-analysis of propafenone, the incidence of recurrent AF was 55.4% (51.3–59.7%) at 6 months and 56.8% (52.3–61.3%) at 1 year (Reimold et al. 1998). All-cause mortality associated with propafenone was 0.3%. Both agents are available in modified-release formulations (propafenone SR and flecainide XL). Because of the danger of organization of AF into atrial

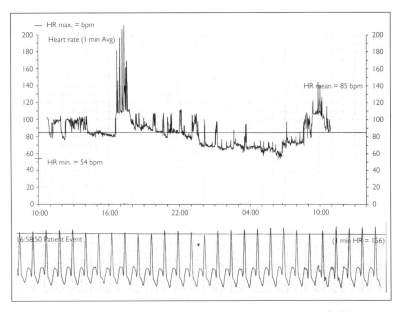

Figure 5.6 Twenty-four-hour tachogram (top panel) of a patient with paroxysmal atrial fibrillation treated with flecainide 100 mg twice daily. The recurrent atrial arrhythmia is atrial flutter rather than fibrillation and there are periods of 1:1 or 2:1 atrioventricular conduction (bottom panel). Co-administration of an atrioventricular nodal blocking drug is essential to prevent high ventricular rates.

flutter with 1:1 or 2:1 conduction (Figure 5.6), concomitant use of AV slowing agents such as beta-blockers and non-dihydropyridine calcium channel blockers are recommended.

5.4.4 **Sotalol**

Sotalol is a modestly effective and safe prophylactic antiarrhythmic drug in patients with AF and stable coronary artery disease in the absence of previous myocardial infarction and left ventricular systolic dysfunction, and patients with hypertension without evidence of left ventricular hypertrophy. Because of its beta-blocking effect, sotalol offers the additional benefit of ventricular rate slowing during recurrences (Benditt et al. 1999).

However, in CTAF (Canadian Trial of Atrial Fibrillation), sotalol was significantly inferior to amiodarone for the long-term maintenance of sinus rhythm (37% vs 65%) (Roy et al. 2000). In SAFE-T (Sotalol Amiodarone Atrial Fibrillation Efficacy Trial), sotalol was also less effective than amiodarone post cardioversion for persistent AF (the median time to a recurrence was 6 days on placebo, 74 days of sotalol, and 487 days on amiodarone) (Singh et al. 2005). At 2 years, approximately 30% of patients treated with sotalol remained in sinus rhythm compared with 60% of patients on amiodarone and 10% of patients on placebo. The efficacy of sotalol was similar to that of class I antiarrhythmic drugs and inferior to that of amiodarone in the AFFIRM substudy (48%, 45%, and 66%, respectively) (The AFFIRM First Antiarrhythmic Drug Substudy Investigators 2003).

Hypotension and bradycardia are the most common cardiovascular adverse effects of sotalol with the incidence of 6–10%. Proarrhythmias associated with QT interval prolongation were observed in 1–4% of patients, usually within 72 hours after the first dose.

5.4.5 **Dofetilide**

Unlike propafenone, flecainide, and sotalol, dofetilide is safe to use in patients with previous myocardial infarction and/or heart failure. In the DIAMOND (Danish Investigations of Arrhythmia and Mortality ON Dofetilide) AF substudy of DIAMOND-CHF and DIAMOND-MI trials, 506 patients with AF at baseline were more likely to remain in sinus rhythm on treatment with dofetilide 500 mcg twice daily compared with placebo (79% vs 42%) (Pedersen et al. 2001).

In the dose-ranging SAFIRE-D (Symptomatic Atrial Fibrillation Investigative Research on Dofetilide) study of 325 patients with persistent AF or flutter for 2–26 weeks, dofetilide exhibited a dose-related effect: 40%, 37%, and 58% patients receiving 250, 500, and 1000 mcg of dofetilide, respectively, were in sinus rhythm after 1 year compared with 25% in the placebo group (Singh et al. 2000).

The major safety concern about dofetilide is its torsadogenic potential which is dose related and often occurs within the first 48–72 hours after the start of treatment in up to 3.3% of patients. This made the in-hospital initiation of dofetilide mandatory.

5.4.6 **Amiodarone**

The potential of amiodarone to maintain sinus rhythm in patients with AF and a relative cardiac safety in patients with significant structural heart disease has been repeatedly shown in observational and prospective, randomized, controlled studies. Data from the CHF-STAT (Congestive Heart Failure Survival Trial of Antiarrhythmic Therapy) substudy showed that patients who received amiodarone had fewer recurrences of AF and were twice as less likely to develop new AF compared with placebo (Deedwania et al. 1998). The safety of amiodarone was indirectly demonstrated in the AF-CHF study (Roy et al. 2008).

Amiodarone has a low torsadogenic potential (< 1%). Given its neutral effect on all-cause mortality, amiodarone should be considered a drug of choice for management of AF in patients with congestive heart failure, hypertrophic cardiomyopathy, and hypertension with significant left ventricular hypertrophy. However, there was a warning from the recent subgroup analysis of SCD-HeFT (SCD-Sudden Cardiac Death in Heart Failure Trial) which has suggested that amiodarone was associated with excess mortality in patients with NYHA class III heart failure (Bardy et al. 2005).

5.4.7 **Dronedarone**

The antiarrhythmic potential of dronedarone has been studied in two high-quality, medium-size efficacy and safety trials. The EURIDIS (EURopean trial In atrial fibrillation or flutter patients receiving Dronedarone for the maIntenance of Sinus rhythm) and its American-Australian-African equivalent ADONIS, have shown that dronedarone was superior to placebo in prevention of recurrent paroxysmal and persistent AF and was also effective in controlling ventricular rates (Singh et al. 2007).

A simultaneously running study, ANDROMEDA (ANtiarrhythmic trial with DROnedarone in Moderate to severe heart failure Evaluating morbidity DecreAse), in patients with severe congestive heart failure was stopped prematurely after 627 patients out of the 1000 planned were enrolled, because an interim safety analysis revealed an excess of deaths in the dronedarone arm compared with placebo (8% vs 13.8%; hazard ratio 2.13, 95% confidence interval, 1.07–4.25; p = 0.027) (Køber et al. 2008). Although ANDROMEDA clearly defined a population that should not receive dronedarone, it had done little else to clarify the safety profile of the drug. The study only included about 25–30% of patients with AF and was chiefly the study in patients with advanced or recently decompensated heart failure.

The post hoc analysis of the EURIDIS and ADONIS studies showed that patients treated with dronedarone had a 27% reduction in relative risk of hospitalization for cardiovascular causes and death (22.8% vs 30.9% on placebo) (Singh et al. 2007). Subsequently, the ATHENA (A placebo controlled, double blind Trial to assess the efficacy of dronedarone for the prevention of cardiovascular Hospitalization or death from any cause in patiENts with Atrial fibrillation and flutter) trial in 4628 high-risk patients has demonstrated that therapy with dronedarone prolonged time to first cardiovascular hospitalization or death from any cause (the composite primary endpoint) by 24% compared with placebo (Hohnloser et al. 2008). This effect was driven by the reduction in cardiovascular hospitalizations (25%), particularly hospitalizations for AF (37%). All-cause mortality was similar in the dronedarone and placebo groups (5% and 6%, respectively); however, dronedarone significantly reduced deaths from cardiovascular causes.

In the ATHENA study, there were 473 patients who seemed to remain in AF throughout the study. A retrospective analysis of these patients showed that fewer of these patients were in the dronedarone group (178 vs 295), and that those treated with dronedarone had a similar reduction of the primary ATHENA endpoint (hazard ratio = 0.76) as for the trial population in general (Nieuwlaat et al. 2011). Subsequently, the PALLAS (Permanent Atrial fibriLLAtion outcome Study) in patients with permanent AF and risk factors was instigated, but was stopped prematurely due to excess of adverse events in the dronedarone arm (Connolly et al. 2011).

The results contrasted markedly with those of ATHENA. The stroke and death rates were approximately double in the dronedarone group compared with placebo. The major difference between PALLAS and ATHENA was that the patients in PALLAS were very largely in long-standing permanent AF, whereas the majority of patients in ATHENA had recurrent forms of AF and many were in sinus rhythm for the majority of the trial. Any advantage from achieving sinus rhythm was not possible in PALLAS (Camm and Savelieva 2013).

Therefore, dronedarone is currently recommended for reducing the need for hospitalization for cardiovascular events in patients with paroxysmal AF or after conversion

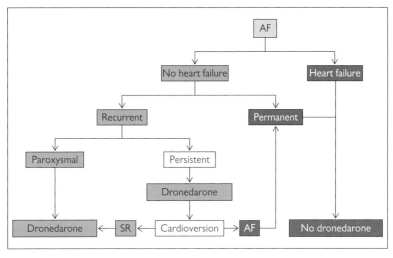

Figure 5.7 Clinical algorithm for deciding whether treatment with dronedarone is appropriate. AF = atrial fibrillation; SR = sinus rhythm.

of persistent AF, but should not be used in patients with permanent AF or advanced or recently decompensated heart failure (Figure 5.7).

5.4.8 **Ranolazine**

Recently, ranolazine, an antianginal agent, which selectively inhibits several ion channels with a preferential effect at the atrial level (Verrier et al. 2012), has demonstrated a promising antiarrhythmic potential for facilitating electrical cardioversion in refractory patients (Murdock et al. 2012), enhancing pharmacological cardioversion while acting synergistically with amiodarone (Fragakis et al. 2012), and also showing the efficacy as a 'pill-in-the-pocket' approach (Murdock et al. 2008) including patients with structural heart disease. The drug has recently been investigated for prevention of recurrent AF post cardioversion and for suppression of paroxysmal AF in combination with dronedarone. Two randomized studies of ranolazine were present at the late breaking trials session during the Heart Rhythm Society meeting in May 2014. The RAFFAELLO (Ranolazine in Atrial Fibrillation Following An ELectricaL CardiOversion) tested the efficacy of several escalating doses of ranolazine against placebo in preventing recurrent persistent AF following electrical cardioversion in 241 patients. The recurrence rates of AF at 4 weeks of treatment in placebo, ranolazine 375 mg bd, ranolazine 500 mg bd, and ranolazine 750 mg bd were in 56.4%, 56.9%, 41.7%, and 39.7%, respectively. When combined, the two higher doses were significantly more effective than the lowest dose or placebo in preventing recurrent AF. In the HARMONY (A Study to Evaluate the Effect of Ranolazine and Dronedarone When Given Alone and in Combination in Patients With Paroxysmal Atrial Fibrillation) trial which enrolled 134 patients with permanent pacemakers, explored the efficacy of various combinations of ranolazine and dronedarone (typically at lower doses than recommended for each individual drug). Compared with placebo, the group receiving ranolazine 750 mg bd and dronedarone 225 bd mg had a greater percentage change in AF burden from baseline to 12 weeks. Further larger studies with ranolazine are planned.

5.5 Optimizing the use of antiarrhythmic drugs: special situations

5.5.1 Shortening the duration of therapy

Systematic reviews of antiarrhythmic drug treatment in AF present convincing evidence of efficacy, but also underscore a non-negligible risk of adverse effects and increased mortality (Figure 5.8) (Freemantle et al. 2011; Lafuente-Lafuente et al. 2012). One solution is restriction of dose and duration of treatment. The argument for this approach is that if antiarrhythmic drugs are prescribed for a few weeks after cardioversion, sufficient time would be available for reverse atrial electrical remodelling, and that recurrence would then be unlikely even when the antiarrhythmic drug was no longer used.

Only a few trials explored this option. The Flec-SL (Flecainide Short Long) trial in 635 patients has shown that short-term antiarrhythmic drug therapy limited to 4 weeks after cardioversion conveyed a slightly lesser, but still significant antiarrhythmic effect on recurrence of AF, estimated at 80% of the effect of traditional long-term therapy over the first 6 months after cardioversion (Kirchhof et al. 2012). The duration of follow-up was short, and it is likely that long-term treatment might be necessary because reversal of the electrophysiological effects of a fast atrial rhythm will not counteract changes due to underlying structural heart disease, autonomic aberration, or inflammatory or toxic effects that induced AF in the first place (Camm and Savelieva 2012). In another trial, episodic amiodarone was not nearly as effective as continuous amiodarone in terms of a composite primary outcome containing efficacy and safety events (Ahmed et al. 2008).

Hence, these trials suggest that short-term antiarrhythmic drug therapy after cardioversion should not be the default type of treatment and should not be considered with amiodarone, but may be useful in patients who are either at high risk for drug-induced adverse effects or for patients with a low likelihood of recurrent AF.

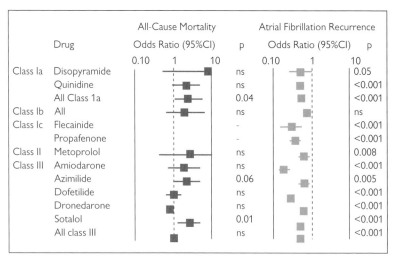

CI, confidence interval.

Figure 5.8 Systematic review of the effects of antiarrhythmic drugs on all-cause mortality and recurrence of atrial fibrillation following cardioversion.

5.5.2 'Pill-in-the-pocket' approach

In some patients with no or minimal structural heart disease and relatively infrequent (< 12 per year), symptomatic paroxysms of AF of distinct onset, a single oral loading dose of propafenone (450–600 mg) or flecainide (200–300 mg) can be used for termination of AF outside the hospital setting. The drug is only taken at the time of arrhythmia rather than on a regular basis, and long-term exposure is avoided, while side effects are minimized. In clinical trials, AF terminated in 50–60% patients at 3 hours and 70–80% patients at 8 hours following the ingestion of a single oral loading dose of propafenone or flecainide compared with 18% and 39% on placebo (Khan 2001, 2003).

In a proof-of-concept study in a selected cohort of 210 patients who had been successfully treated in-hospital with either oral flecainide or propafenone for paroxysmal AF, a single oral dose taken within 5 minutes of noticing palpitations was associated with a termination of AF and an almost tenfold reduction in the monthly number of visits to emergency departments (Alboni et al 2004).

It is mandatory that the efficacy and safety of this strategy is first tested in-hospital and is generally recommended that patients should not be taking a prophylactic antiarrhythmic drug (Camm and Savelieva 2007). There is always the danger of development of atrial flutter with 1:1 AV conduction, and the concomitant administration of an AV blocking agent is advocated in some cases. Long-term anticoagulation is required in high-risk individuals. The experience with this strategy is limited, and it is unknown how valuable it will be in the long term because AF tends to progress over time.

5.6 Upstream therapy

Treatment of the underlying heart disease that is commonly associated with AF, such as hypertension and heart failure, does not only improve major cardiovascular outcomes and survival in patients with AF, but can also deter the occurrence of new AF or, acting synergistically with specific rhythm control therapies, reduce the likelihood of recurrent AF. Such agents may include beta-blockers, which have very modest antiarrhythmic properties, and traditionally non-antiarrhythmic drugs, such as angiotensin-converting enzyme (ACE) inhibitors, angiotensin receptor blockers, statins, and fish oil supplements.

One of the examples is lower stroke rates in the warfarin arms of contemporary stroke prevention trials compared with historic warfarin-treated cohorts, reflecting better management of hypertension and risk factors. Similarly, the results of the AF-CHF trial which did not find AF predictive of cardiovascular death, likely reflect an improvement in the management of heart failure compared with the earlier heart failure studies which, in contrast, identified a twofold increase in mortality associated with AF than sinus rhythm (Dries et al. 1998).

Newer therapies also improved major cardiovascular outcomes in some AF patients compared with older drugs. Thus, in the LIFE (Losartan Intervention for Endpoint reduction in hypertension) study in patients with left ventricular hypertrophy, the incidence of cardiovascular death, stroke, and myocardial infarction was reduced by 42% with the losartan-based therapy compared with atenolol (Wachtell et al. 2005). In the post hoc analysis of the ACTIVE I (Atrial fibrillation Clopidogrel Trial with Irbesartan for prevention of Vascular Events – Irbesartan), there was a modest, but statistically significant, reduction in the composite of stroke, transient ischaemic attacks, and systemic embolism by 13% and a 40% reduction in primary haemorrhagic stroke and secondary transformation of ischaemic stroke with irbesartan compared with placebo, probably as a result of a lower blood pressure (Yusuf et al. 2011).

The concept of upstream therapies is appealing because these therapies target both the formation and evolution of the substrate for AF (Kourliouros et al. 2009). These agents may have the antiarrhythmic potential, additional to any treatment effect on the underlying disease, for example, targeting structural changes in the atria, such as fibrosis, hypertrophy, inflammation, and oxidative stress, or even exerting the direct effects on atrial ion channels, gap junctions, and calcium handling.

Retrospective analyses and reports from the studies in which AF was a pre-specified secondary endpoint, have shown a sustained reduction in new-onset AF with ACE inhibitors and angiotensin receptor blockers in patients with significant underlying heart disease and in the incidence of AF after cardiac surgery in patients treated with statins (Savelieva et al. 2011a). In the LIFE study, a reduction in the left atrial size on treatment was associated with a 79% lower risk of new-onset AF (Wachtell et al. 2010).

However, in the secondary prevention setting, the results with upstream therapies are significantly less encouraging, with the majority of large prospective randomized clinical trials yielding controversial, mostly negative, results. Neither ACE inhibitors and angiotensin receptor blockers, nor statins or fish oil supplements have been demonstrated to prevent recurrent paroxysmal or persistent AF (Savelieva et al. 2011b).

5.7 **Ablation**

Interventional techniques are highly effective therapies for patients who remain symptomatic despite optimal medical therapy.

5.7.1 **AV nodal ablation**

If the heart rate cannot be adequately controlled the proximal AV conduction system can be destroyed, usually with radiofrequency energy or cryotherapy. After this destructive procedure the ventricular rate must be supported using an artificial pacemaker. Usually it is not necessary to use an AV pacemaker if the patient is in permanent AF, but it is needed if the AF is intermittent. Since patients are paced for prolonged continuous periods after AV node/His bundle ablation it is often essential to pace both the left and right ventricles (biventricular pacing) to avoid or manage left ventricular dysfunction optimally, especially in those with already depressed left ventricular function. For a limited period (1–3 months) after the ablation procedure it is usual to pace at a faster rate (~100 bpm) over several weeks or months and subsequently reduce the lower pacing rate limit to 70 bpm or less.

This procedure is remarkably effective, and is suitable for older patients, but should generally be avoided in the young if alternative strategies such as left atrial ablation are available.

5.7.2 **Left atrial ablation**

If antiarrhythmic drugs fail to prevent the symptomatic recurrences of intermittent AF, particularly when several drugs alone and in combination have been tried, it is useful to undertake left atrial ablation, usually pulmonary vein isolation. This is a relatively straightforward technique, with high efficacy and a low but still measurable complication rate, when skilled operators perform the procedure. It is most effective when the atria are small, the left ventricle functions normally, and underlying cardiovascular disease and other major co-morbidities are not present. Transthoracic echocardiography should be performed to assess patients prior to referral. In most centres a period of effective anticoagulation (for at least 3 weeks) is recommended prior to the ablation procedure, especially if the patient has frequent or long duration relapses of the arrhythmia.

A major consideration is whether to offer left atrial ablation early in the progress of the disease (prior to multiple or any failure of antiarrhythmic drug treatment) on the basis that less atrial remodelling (fibrosis, dilation, etc.) will have taken place and the major therapeutic target is the isolation of triggers to AF (relatively easy) rather than modification of the AF substrate (relatively difficult). This may be considered in very good centres.

Early complications include pericardial haemorrhage, tamponade (not unusual), stroke (uncommon) and atrio-oesophageal fistula (rare). Later complications include the occurrence of atrial tachycardias caused by the procedure (often left atrial), and recurrences of the AF that has not been successfully eliminated by the procedure. Generally, early arrhythmias are managed conservatively and repeat ablation, which is often needed, is delayed until at least 3 months following the procedure. The choice of antiarrhythmic drug therapy follows the usual guideline. Anticoagulation is necessary for at least 3 months following the procedure since the risk of thromboembolism is related not only to atrial arrhythmia but also to the endothelial damage produced by the procedure. Subsequent anticoagulation strategy depends on the thromboembolic risk as assessed, for example, by the $CHADS_2$ or CHA_2DS_2-VASc scores.

When symptomatic recurrences occur after an ablation procedure antiarrhythmic drug therapy may be needed and it is not unusual that drugs that were ineffective prior to ablation may then be successful. This may be because the mechanism of the post-ablation arrhythmia is different or because the triggers are more vulnerable or the substrate is less resistant.

5.8 Conclusion

The therapy of AF requires a range of therapeutic options of which antiarrhythmic drugs are an important component. Only a limited number of agents are now available and their use must be carefully considered and controlled. The major indication is symptomatic arrhythmia and the choice of drug depends largely on safety considerations. In patients with minimal or no heart disease any agent may be considered but it is usual to try beta blockade, flecainide or propafenone, sotalol or dronedarone, and amiodarone or dofetilide in that order. When left ventricular hypertrophy is present only amiodarone, and possibly dronedarone, are appropriate. In patients with coronary heart disease, sotalol, dronedarone, and amiodarone may be tried and when there is significant heart failure only dofetilide or amiodarone can be used. In studies that compare efficacy of these agents amiodarone is demonstrably the most effective and other drugs seem to be equipotent but may be effective in different patients. As yet there is little way to predict effectiveness of a particular agent. If AF recurs after cardiac ablation antiarrhythmic drugs may be successful even when ineffective prior to ablation. All patients with recurrent episodes of AF must be considered for rate control even when a rhythm control is the primary strategy.

References

Ahmed S, Rienstra M, Crijns HJ, Links TP, Wiesfeld AC, Hillege HL, *et al.* Continuous vs. episodic prophylactic treatment with amiodarone for the prevention of atrial fibrillation: a randomized trial. *JAMA* 2008; 300: 1784–92.

Alboni P, Botto GL, Baldi N, Luzi M, Russo V, Gianfranchi L, *et al.* Outpatient treatment of recent-onset atrial fibrillation with the 'pill-in-the-pocket' approach. *N Engl J Med* 2004; 351: 2384–91.

Bardy GH, Lee KL, Mark DB, Poole JE, Packer DL, Boineau R, *et al.* Amiodarone or an implantable cardioverter-defibrillator for congestive heart failure. *N Engl J Med* 2005; 352: 225–37.

Benditt DG, Williams JH, Jin J, Deering TF, Zucker R, Browne K, *et al.* Maintenance of sinus rhythm with oral d,l-sotalol therapy in patients with symptomatic atrial fibrillation and/or atrial flutter. *Am J Cardiol* 1999; 84: 270–7.

Brignole M, Auricchio A, Baron-Esquivias G, Bordachar P, Boriani G, Breithardt OA, *et al.* 2013 ESC guidelines on cardiac pacing and cardiac resynchronization therapy: the task force on cardiac pacing and resynchronization therapy of the European Society of Cardiology (ESC). Developed in collaboration with the European Heart Rhythm Association (EHRA). *Europace* 2013; 15: 1070–118.

Camm AJ. Safety considerations in the pharmacological management of atrial fibrillation. *Int J Cardiol* 2008; 127: 299–306.

Camm AJ, Kirchhof P, Lip GY, Schotten U, Savelieva I, Ernst S, *et al.* Guidelines for the management of atrial fibrillation: the Task Force for the Management of Atrial Fibrillation of the European Society of Cardiology (ESC). *Europace* 2010; 12: 1360–420.

Camm AJ, Savelieva I. Some patients with paroxysmal atrial fibrillation should carry flecainide or propafenone to self treat. *BMJ* 2007; 334: 637.

Camm AJ, Savelieva I. The long and short of antiarrhythmic drug treatment. *Lancet* 2012; 380: 198–200.

Camm AJ, Savelieva I. Dronedarone for the treatment of non-permanent atrial fibrillation: National Institute for Health and Clinical Excellence guidance. *Heart* 2013; 99: 1476–80.

Capucci A, Villani GQ, Aschieri D, Rosi A, Piepoli MF. Oral amiodarone increases the efficacy of direct-current cardioversion in restoration of sinus rhythm in patients with chronic atrial fibrillation. *Eur Heart J* 2000; 21: 66–73.

Chimienti M, Cullen MT Jr, Casadei G. Safety of long-term flecainide and propafenone in the management of patients with symptomatic paroxysmal atrial fibrillation: report from the Flecainide And Propafenone Italian Study Investigators. *Am J Cardiol* 1996; 77: 60A–75A.

Connolly SJ, Camm AJ, Halperin JL, Joyner C, Alings M, Amerena J, *et al.* Dronedarone in high-risk permanent atrial fibrillation. *N Engl J Med* 2011; 365: 2268–76.

Corley SD, Epstein AE, DiMarco JP, Domanski MJ, Geller N, Greene HL, *et al.* Relationships between sinus rhythm, treatment, and survival in the Atrial Fibrillation Follow-Up Investigation of Rhythm Management (AFFIRM) Study. *Circulation* 2004; 109: 1509–13.

Cosio FG, Aliot E, Botto GL, Heidbüchel H, Geller CJ, Kirchhof P, *et al.* Delayed rhythm control of atrial fibrillation may be a cause of failure to prevent recurrences: reasons for change to active antiarrhythmic treatment at the time of the first detected episode. *Europace* 2008; 10: 21–7.

Crijns HJ, Gosselink AT, Lie KI. Propafenone versus disopyramide for maintenance of sinus rhythm after electrical cardioversion of atrial fibrillation: a randomized, double-blind study. PRODIS Study Group. *Cardiovasc Drugs Ther* 1996; 10: 145–52.

De Vos CB, Breithardt G, Camm AJ, Dorian P, Kowey PR, Le Heuzey JY, *et al.* Progression of atrial fibrillation in the REgistry on Cardiac rhythm disORDers assessing the control of Atrial Fibrillation cohort: clinical correlates and the effect of rhythm-control therapy. *Am Heart J* 2012; 163: 887–93.

De Vos CB, Pisters R, Nieuwlaat R, Prins MH, Tieleman RG, Coelen RJ, *et al.* Progression from paroxysmal to persistent atrial fibrillation clinical correlates and prognosis. *J Am Coll Cardiol* 2010; 55: 725–31.

Deedwania PC, Singh BN, Ellenbogen K, Fisher S, Fletcher R, Singh SN; for the Department of Veterans Affairs CHF-STAT Investigators. Spontaneous conversion and maintenance of sinus rhythm by amiodarone in patients with heart failure and atrial fibrillation: observations from the Veterans Affairs Congestive Heart Failure Survival Trial of Antiarrhythmic Therapy (CHF-STAT). *Circulation* 1998; 98: 2574–9.

Dries DL, Exner DV, Gersh BJ, Domanski MJ, Waclawiw MA, Stevenson LV. Atrial fibrillation is associated with an increased risk for mortality and heart failure progression in patients with asymptomatic and symptomatic left ventricular systolic dysfunction: a retrospective analysis of the SOLVD trials. Studies Of Left Ventricular Dysfunction. *J Am Coll Cardiol* 1998; 32: 695–703.

Echt DS, Liebson PR, Mitchell LB, Peters RW, Obias-Manno D, Barker AH, *et al.* Mortality and morbidity in patients receiving encainide, flecainide, or placebo. The Cardiac Arrhythmia Suppression Trial. *N Engl J Med* 1991; 324: 781–8.

Farshi R, Kistner D, Sarma JS, Longmate JA, Singh BN. Ventricular rate control in chronic atrial fibrillation during daily activity and programmed exercise: a crossover open-label study of five drug regimens. *J Am Coll Cardiol* 1999; 33: 304–10.

Fragakis N, Koskinas KC, Katritsis DG, Pagourelias ED, Zografos T, Geleris P. Comparison of effectiveness of ranolazine plus amiodarone versus amiodarone alone for conversion of recent-onset atrial fibrillation. *Am J Cardiol* 2012; 110: 673–7.

Freemantle N, Lafuente-Lafuente C, Mitchell S, Eckert L, Reynolds M. Mixed treatment comparison of dronedarone, amiodarone, sotalol, flecainide, and propafenone, for the management of atrial fibrillation. *Europace* 2011; 13: 329–45.

Hohnloser SH, Connolly SJ, Crijns HJ, Page RL, Seiz W, Torp-Petersen C. Rationale and design of ATHENA: A placebo-controlled, double-blind, parallel arm Trial to assess the efficacy of dronedarone 400 mg bid for the prevention of cardiovascular Hospitalization or death from any cause in patiENts with Atrial fibrillation/atrial flutter. *J Cardiovasc Electrophysiol* 2008; 19: 69–73.

Jahangir A, Lee V, Friedman PA, Trusty JM, Hodge DO, Kopecky SL, et al. Long-term progression and outcomes with aging in patients with lone atrial fibrillation: a 30-year follow-up study. *Circulation* 2007; 115: 3050–6.

Karlson BW, Torstensson I, Abjörn C, Jansson SO, Peterson LE. Disopyramide in the maintenance of sinus rhythm after electroconversion of atrial fibrillation. A placebo-controlled one-year follow-up study. *Eur Heart J* 1988; 9: 284–90.

Katritsis DG, Panagiotakos DB, Karvouni E, Giazitzoglou E, Korovesis S, Paxinos G, et al. Comparison of effectiveness of carvedilol versus bisoprolol for maintenance of sinus rhythm after cardioversion of persistent atrial fibrillation. *Am J Cardiol* 2003; 92: 1116–19.

Kerr CR, Humphries KH, Talajic M, Klein GJ, Connolly SJ, Green M, et al. Progression to chronic atrial fibrillation after the initial diagnosis of paroxysmal atrial fibrillation: results from the Canadian Registry of Atrial Fibrillation. *Am Heart J* 2005; 149: 489–96.

Khan IA. Single oral loading dose of propafenone for pharmacological cardioversion of recent-onset atrial fibrillation. *J Am Coll Cardiol* 2001; 37: 542–7.

Khan IA. Oral loading single dose flecainide for pharmacological cardioversion of recent-onset atrial fibrillation. *Int J Cardiol* 2003; 87: 121–8.

Khand AU, Rankin AC, Martin W, Taylor J, Gemmell I, Cleland JG. Carvedilol alone or in combination with digoxin for the management of atrial fibrillation in patients with heart failure? *J Am Coll Cardiol* 2003; 42: 1944–51.

Kirchhof P, Andresen D, Bosch R, Borggrefe M, Meinertz T, Parade U, et al. Short-term versus long-term antiarrhythmic drug treatment after cardioversion of atrial fibrillation (Flec-SL): a prospective, randomised, open-label, blinded endpoint assessment trial. *Lancet* 2012; 380: 238–46.

Køber L, Torp-Pedersen C, McMurray JJ, Gøtzsche O, Lévy S, Crijns H, et al. Increased mortality after dronedarone therapy for severe heart failure. *N Engl J Med* 2008; 358: 2678–87.

Kourliouros A, Savelieva I, Kiotsekoglou A, Jahangir M, Camm J. Current concepts in the pathogenesis of atrial fibrillation. *Am Heart J* 2009; 157: 243–52.

Kühlkamp V, Schirdewan A, Stangl K, Homberg M, Ploch M, Beck OA. Use of metoprolol CR/XL to maintain sinus rhythm after conversion from persistent atrial fibrillation: a randomized, double-blind, placebo-controlled study. *J Am Coll Cardiol* 2000; 36: 139–46.

Lafuente-Lafuente C, Longas-Tejero MA, Bergmann JF, Belmin J. Antiarrhythmics for maintaining sinus rhythm after cardioversion of atrial fibrillation. *Cochrane Database Syst Rev* 2012; 5: CD005049.

Lewis RV, Irvine N, McDevitt DG. Relationships between heart rate, exercise tolerance and cardiac output in atrial fibrillation: the effects of treatment with digoxin, verapamil and diltiazem. *Eur Heart J* 1988; 9: 777–81.

Murdock DK, Kersten M, Kaliebe J, Larrain G. The use of oral ranolazine to convert new or paroxysmal atrial fibrillation: a review of experience with implications for possible "pill in the pocket" approach to atrial fibrillation. *Indian Pacing Electrophysiol J* 2008; 9: 260–7.

Murdock DK, Reiffel JA, Kaliebe JW, Larrain G. The use of ranolazine to facilitate electrical cardioversion in cardioversion-resistant patients: a case series. *Pacing Clin Electrophysiol* 2012; 35: 302v7.

Nieuwlaat R, Hohnloser SH, Connolly SJ. Effect of dronedarone in patients with permanent atrial fibrillation during the ATHENA study. *Eur Heart J* 2011; 32(Suppl): 618.

Olshansky B, Rosenfeld LE, Warner AL, Solomon AJ, O'Neill G, Sharma A, et al. The Atrial Fibrillation Follow-up Investigation of Rhythm Management (AFFIRM) study: approaches to control rate in atrial fibrillation. *J Am Coll Cardiol* 2004; 43: 1201–8.

Pedersen OD, Bagger H, Keller N, Marchant B, Kober L, Torp-Pedersen C. Efficacy of dofetilide in the treatment of atrial fibrillation-flutter in patients with reduced left ventricular function. A Danish Investigations of Arrhythmia and Mortality ON Dofetilide (DIAMOND) Substudy. *Circulation* 2001; 104: 292–6.

Plewan A, Lehmann G, Ndrepepa G, Schreieck J, Alt EU, Schömig A, Schmitt C. Maintenance of sinus rhythm after electrical cardioversion of persistent atrial fibrillation: sotalol vs bisoprolol. *Eur Heart J* 2001; 22: 1504–10.

Rawles JM. What is meant by a 'controlled' ventricular rate in atrial fibrillation? *Br Heart J* 1990; 63: 157–61.

Reimold SC, Maisel WH, Antman EM. Propafenone for the treatment of supraventricular tachycardia and atrial fibrillation: a meta-analysis. *Am J Cardiol* 1998; 82: 66N–71N.

Roy D, Talajic M, Dorian P, Connolly S, Eisenberg MJ, Green M, *et al.* Amiodarone to prevent recurrence of atrial fibrillation. *N Engl J Med* 2000; 342: 913–20.

Roy D, Talajic M, Nattel S, Wyse DG, Dorian P, Lee KL, *et al.* Rhythm control versus rate control for atrial fibrillation and heart failure. *N Engl J Med* 2008; 358: 2667–77.

Savelieva I, Camm AJ. Clinical relevance of silent atrial fibrillation: prevalence, prognosis, quality of life, and management. *J Interv Card Electrophysiol* 2000; 4: 369–82.

Savelieva I, Kakouros N, Kourliouros A, Camm AJ. Upstream therapies for management of atrial fibrillation: review of clinical evidence and implications for European Society of Cardiology guidelines. Part I: primary prevention. *Europace* 2011a; 13: 308–28.

Savelieva I, Kakouros N, Kourliouros A, Camm AJ. Upstream therapies for management of atrial fibrillation: review of clinical evidence and implications for European Society of Cardiology guidelines. Part II: secondary prevention. *Europace* 2011b; 13: 610–25.

Singh BN, Connolly SJ, Crijns HJ, Roy D, Kowey PR, Capucci A, *et al.* Dronedarone for maintenance of sinus rhythm in atrial fibrillation or flutter. *N Engl J Med* 2007; 357: 987–99.

Singh BN, Singh SN, Reda DJ, Tang XC, Lopez B, Harris CL, *et al.* Amiodarone versus sotalol for atrial fibrillation. *N Engl J Med* 2005; 352: 1861–72.

Singh S, Zoble RG, Yellen L Brodsky MA, Feld GK, Berk M, *et al.* Efficacy and safety of oral dofetilide in converting to and maintaining sinus rhythm in patients with chronic atrial fibrillation or atrial flutter: the Symptomatic Atrial Fibrillation Investigative Research on Dofetilide (SAFIRE-D) Study. *Circulation* 2000; 102: 2385–90.

Talajic M, Khairy P, Levesque S, Connolly SJ, Dorian P, Dubuc M, *et al.* Maintenance of sinus rhythm and survival in patients with heart failure and atrial fibrillation. *J Am Coll Cardiol* 2010; 55: 1796–802.

The AFFIRM First Antiarrhythmic Drug Substudy Investigators. Maintenance of sinus rhythm in patients with atrial fibrillation: an AFFIRM Substudy of First Antiarrhythmic Drug. *J Am Coll Cardiol* 2003; 42: 20–9.

Van Gelder IC, Groenveld HF, Crijns HJ, Tuininga YS, Tijssen JG, Alings AM, *et al.* Lenient versus strict rate control in patients with atrial fibrillation. *N Engl J Med* 2010; 362: 1363–73.

Van Gelder IC, Hagens VE, Bosker HA, Kingma JH, Kamp O, Kingma T, *et al.* A comparison of rate control and rhythm control in patients with recurrent persistent atrial fibrillation. *N Engl J Med* 2002; 347: 1834–40.

Van Gelder IC, Wyse DG, Chandler ML, Cooper HA, Olshansky B, Hagens VE, *et al.* Does intensity of rate-control influence outcome in atrial fibrillation? An analysis of pooled data from the RACE and AFFIRM studies. *Europace* 2006; 8: 935–42.

Verrier RL, Kumar K, Nieminen T, Belardinelli L. Mechanisms of ranolazine's dual protection against atrial and ventricular fibrillation. *Europace* 2012; 15: 317–24.

Wachtell K, Gerdts E, Aurigemma GP, Boman K, Dahlöf B, Nieminen MS, *et al.* In-treatment reduced left atrial diameter during antihypertensive treatment is associated with reduced new-onset atrial fibrillation in hypertensive patients with left ventricular hypertrophy: The LIFE Study. *Blood Press* 2010; 19: 169–75.

Wachtell K, Hornestam B, Lehto M, Slotwiner DJ, Gerdts E, Olsen MH, *et al.* Cardiovascular morbidity and mortality in hypertensive patients with a history of atrial fibrillation: the Losartan Intervention For End Point Reduction in Hypertension (LIFE) study. *J Am Coll Cardiol* 2005; 45: 705–11.

Whitbeck MG, Charnigo RJ, Khairy P, Ziada K, Bailey AL, Zegarra MM, *et al.* Increased mortality among patients taking digoxin – analysis from the AFFIRM study. *Eur Heart J* 2013; 34: 1481–8.

Wyse DG, Waldo AL, DiMarco JP, Domanski MJ, Rosenberg Y, Schron EB, *et al.* A comparison of rate control and rhythm control in patients with atrial fibrillation. *N Engl J Med* 2002; 347: 1825–33.

Yusuf S, Healey JS, Pogue J, Chrolavicius S, Flather M, Hart RG, *et al.* Irbesartan in patients with atrial fibrillation. *N Engl J Med* 2011; 364: 928–38.

Chapter 6

Anticoagulation selection and stroke prevention

Christos Dresios and Gregory Y.H. Lip

> ## Key points
>
> - The landscape of stroke prevention in AF has evolved, with the availability of excellent data from 4 non-vitamin K oral anticoagulants (NOACs).
> - Guidelines now focus on initial identification of 'low risk' patients who do not need any antithrombotic therapy. Subsequent to this step, effective stroke prevention (ie. OAC) can be offered to patients with ≥1 stroke risk factores.
> - Assess stroke risk using the CHA_2DS_2-VASc score, which is now used in international guidelines.
> - Assess bleeding risk using HAS-BLED. A high HAS-BLED score is not a reason to withhold anticoagulation, as the net clinical benefit is even greater in those with high scores.
> - In a de novo AF patient, consider assessing their suitability for VKA using the $SAMe\text{-}TT_2R_2$ score, which would give an informed decision on their likelihood of achieving good quality of INR control, as reflected by a high time in therapeutic range (TTR).

6.1 Epidemiology

Given the fact that many patients suffer from silent atrial fibrillation (AF) and will never present to hospital, the true prevalence of AF probably approaches 2% of the population. AF is increasing in prevalence and incidence and its prevalence is estimated to double in the next 50 years. It is estimated that in the United States up to 16 million people will suffer from AF by 2050. Indeed, the incidence of AF increased by 13% in the past two decades.

Both the incidence and prevalence of AF increases with advancing age and with the presence of cardiovascular disease (Kannel et al. 1982; Krahn et al. 1995; Heeringa et al. 2003). In particular, the prevalence increases from less than 0.5% at 40–50 years, to 5–15% at 80 years. In all age groups, men have a slightly higher incidence of AF than women because the incidence of AF increases dramatically with age and given that women have a greater life expectancy than men, the absolute number of women and men with AF in the elderly is similar (Benjamin et al. 1994; Hnatkova et al. 1998; Kannel et al. 1998; Humphries et al. 2001). When compared to elderly men with AF, elderly women with AF have a significantly elevated risk for stroke, regardless of warfarin use (Avgil Tsadok et al. 2012).

6.2 **Predisposing clinical conditions**

AF is commonly associated with various cardiovascular conditions. The most common predisposing clinical conditions are hypertension, heart failure, and coronary disease.

Epidemiologically, hypertension is one of the most important risk factors associated with AF development by 1.42-fold (Krahn et al. 1995), and furthermore, increases the risk of stroke and other cardiovascular events in patients with AF. Symptomatic heart failure (New York Heart Association (NYHA) classes II–IV) is found in 30–40% of AF patients, and conversely, AF is the most common arrhythmia in patients with heart failure. Thus, heart failure not only can be both a consequence of AF but also a cause of the arrhythmia due to increased atrial pressure and volume overload.

Coronary artery disease is found at least 20% of the AF population (Nieuwlaat et al. 2005; Nabauer et al. 2009). However, it is unclear if uncomplicated coronary artery disease per se represents a risk factor for the development of AF (Goette et al. 2009).

Congenital heart diseases are also correlated with higher risk of AF. For example, AF has been reported in approximately 20% of adults with an atrial septal defect (Tikoff et al. 1968). Cardiomyopathies are also associated with increased risk for AF, especially in young patients (Maron et al. 2006).

Diabetes mellitus is present in 25% of AF patients. Indeed, inadequate control of diabetes mellitus leads to structural remodelling which contributes to the maintenance of AF. Increased left ventricular mass and increased arterial stiffness have been suggested as possible mechanisms (Devereux et al. 2000).

Valvular heart diseases are found in approximately 30% of AF patients (Nieuwlaat et al. 2005; Nabauer et al. 2009). AF appears early in the natural history of mitral stenosis and or regurgitation, whereas it occurs in later stages of aortic valve disease. Rheumatic heart disease, although now uncommon in developed countries, is associated with high incidence of AF in developing countries.

Thyroid dysfunction represents an important predisposing factor for AF and may also predispose to complications related to AF. Obese individuals (body mass index (BMI) > 30 kg/m^2) are significantly more likely to develop AF than those with a normal BMI (< 25 kg/m^2). Indeed, obesity is found in 25% of AF patients (Nabauer et al. 2009) and the mean BMI was 27.5 kg/m^2. Obesity is associated with increased left atrial size and impaired left ventricular diastolic function and these could theoretically lead to an increased AF risk (Stritzke et al. 2009).

Chronic obstructive pulmonary disease (COPD) and AF frequently coexist. Indeed, COPD is present in 10–15% of AF patients, and perhaps represents possibly more a marker for cardiovascular risk in general than a specific predisposing factor for AF. Chronic renal failure is found in 10–15% of AF patients and increases the risk of the development of AF. Various types of surgery are also related to increased risk of AF. Patients undergoing coronary artery bypass graft (CABG) or cardiac valve surgery are at higher risk of developing AF.

Alcohol consumption is also correlated with higher risk of AF. In particular, AF occurs in up to 60% of binge drinkers even without an underlying alcoholic cardiomyopathy (Khan et al. 2013). Most cases of AF occur during and following weekends or holidays after excessive consumption of alcohol. This phenomenon has been termed 'the holiday heart syndrome'.

There may be a causal relationship between obstructive sleep apnoea (OSA) and AF (Kanagala et al. 2003; Schulz et al. 2005). Sleep apnoea, especially in association with other predisposing conditions such us hypertension and diabetes mellitus may be a risk factor for AF due to the fact that apnoea leads to a rise in atrial pressure and volume, or autonomic changes.

All these conditions may also be responsible for the inexorable progression of AF to persistent or permanent forms by promoting anatomical and electric remodelling of the atria which represent the substrate for its maintenance.

6.3 **Complications of atrial fibrillation**

The presence of AF doubles the death rate independently of other known predictors of mortality (Lip et al. 1997; Stewart et al. 2002; Hylek et al. 2003; Lloyd-Jones et al. 2004; Miyasaka et al. 2006; Kirchhof et al. 2007; Naccarelli et al. 2009). Importantly, patients with AF have a fivefold increased risk of stroke when compared to people without AF. Up to 3 million people worldwide have a stroke related to AF each year (Marini et al. 2005; Kannel et al. 2008). The absolute annual risk of stroke in patients with AF of all causes is around 5%, but varies with age and the presence of other risk factors (Morley et al. 1996). Of note, approximately 15% of all strokes are associated with AF, and the association increases steadily with age (Lin et al. 1996).

Hospitalizations for AF have increased dramatically (two- to threefold) in recent years (Wattigney et al. 2003), and hospitalizations due to AF account for one-third of all admissions for cardiac arrhythmias (Camm et al. 2010). The main associated reasons are acute coronary syndrome, worsening of heart failure, thromboembolic complications, and acute arrhythmia management.

Left ventricular (LV) dysfunction is associated with an increased risk of AF, but also represents also an important complication in AF patients. Indeed, AF can cause severe, reversible LV dysfunction in patients without structural heart disease (AF-induced cardiomyopathy) and thus should always be considered when patients present with newly recognized congestive heart failure.

In addition, AF had a negative impact on quality of life and exercise capacity. Of note, patients with AF have significantly poorer quality of life compared with healthy controls, the general population, and other patients with coronary heart disease. Furthermore, there is an association between AF, cognitive decline, and dementia (Park et al. 2007; Rastas et al. 2007).

Although AF is responsible for a variety of symptoms, at least one-third of patients report no overt symptoms and are unaware of their arrhythmic condition (Kerr et al. 1996). Silent AF is diagnosed incidentally during routine physical or electrocardiographic examination. In some cases, asymptomatic AF may manifest in the context of AF-related complications. Silent AF still merits consideration for anticoagulation and rate control therapy according to standard criteria.

6.4 **Stroke prevention**

Despite the fact that AF is an independent risk factor for stroke, this risk is not homogenous and depends on the presence or absence of specific risk factors for stroke in AF. Two systematic reviews have addressed the evidence base for stroke risk factors in AF and concluded that prior stroke/transient ischaemic attack (TIA)/thromboembolism, age, hypertension, diabetes, and structural heart disease are important risk factors (Stroke Risk in Atrial Fibrillation Working Group 2007; Hughes and Lip 2008).

In the last few years, several risk-stratification schemes to predict stroke in patients with non-valvular AF were published. A comparison of these risk-stratifications schemes carried out from The Stroke in AF Working Group led to the conclusion that there were substantial, clinically relevant differences among published schemes. Most had only modest predictive value for stroke. The simplest risk assessment scheme is the $CHADS_2$ score (Table 6.1).

Table 6.1 CHADS$_2$ scoring scheme	
Stroke risk in AF	Score
Congestive heart failure	1
Hypertension	1
Age ≥ 75 years	1
Diabetes mellitus	1
Stroke /transient ischaemic attack/thromboembolism	2
Maximum score	6

In this risk assessment scheme 2 points are assigned for a history of stroke or TIA and 1 point each is assigned for age 75 years, a history of hypertension, diabetes, or recent cardiac failure (Gage et al. 2001).

In its original validation, patients were considered as 'low-risk' if they scored 0, 'intermediate-risk' if they score 1–2, and 'high-risk' if they scored 3 or higher. In patients with a CHADS$_2$ score of 2 or more, chronic oral anticoagulant (OAC) therapy with a vitamin K antagonist (VKA) is recommended to achieve an international normalized ratio (INR) target of 2.5.

Nowadays, in patients with a CHADS$_2$ score of 1, OAC is also the preferred therapy. In patients who refuse the use of any OAC, antiplatelet therapy should be considered, whereby the combination of aspirin 75–100 mg and clopidogrel 75 mg daily is the recommended strategy. In patients without risk factors, the preferred treatment is no antithrombotic therapy rather than aspirin (Sato et al. 2006).

Various published analysis highlighted several pitfalls associated with use of the CHADS$_2$ score. Even patients considered at intermediate risk (CHADS$_2$ score = 1) would benefit from OAC over aspirin use (Gorin et al. 2010). In addition, the CHADS$_2$ score does not include additional common stroke risk factors such as female sex, age 65–74 years, and vascular disease in order to have a more comprehensive and integrated risk model.

The recognition that risk for stroke in AF patients is a continuum and the necessity to identify 'truly low-risk' patients led to the development of a risk factor-based approach in order to obtain a more detailed stroke risk assessment.

The CHA$_2$DS$_2$-VASc score represents a risk factor-based approach for patients with non-valvular AF (Lip and Halperin 2010) that more reliably assists the decision to anticoagulate or not (Lip and Halperin 2010; Lip et al. 2010) (Table 6.2).

In the context of the CHA$_2$DS$_2$VASc score, 2 points are assigned for a history of stroke or TIA, or age 75 or older; and 1 point each is assigned for age 65–74 years, a history of hypertension, diabetes, recent cardiac failure, vascular disease (myocardial infarction (MI), complex aortic plaque, and peripheral arterial disease (PAD), including prior revascularization, amputation due to PAD, or angiographic evidence of PAD, etc.), and female sex.

On the other hand, before starting anticoagulation in AF patients at high risk for stroke, individual bleeding risk should also be considered. Bleeding is the most feared adverse effect associated with anticoagulation therapy and is associated with increased mortality and morbidity.

Various bleeding risk assessment scores have been proposed, but until recently have not had wide uptake, due to their complexity. Based on a 'real-world' cohort of 3978 European patients with AF from the EuroHeart Survey, a new simple bleeding risk score was recently

Table 6.2 The CHA$_2$DS$_2$-VASc score for risk of stroke in non-valvular AF	
Risk factor	Score
Congestive cardiac failure	1
Hypertension	1
Age ≥ 75	2
Diabetes mellitus	1
Stroke/transient ischaemic attack/thromboembolism	2
Vascular disease	1
Age 65–74	1
Female sex	1
Maximum score	9

described—the HAS-BLED (hypertension, abnormal renal/liver function, stroke, bleeding history or bleeding tendency, labile INR, elderly (> 65), drugs/alcohol use) score (Table 6.3) (Pisters et al. 2010).

AF patients with a HAS-BLED score of 3 or higher are considered 'high risk' and in such patients, caution and regular follow-up is needed after the initiation of antithrombotic therapy. In addition to that, particular emphasis should be placed on the management of the reversible risk factors which results in the beneficial modification of the individual bleeding risk profile. A high HAS-BLED score per se should not be used to withhold OAC therapy.

Until recently warfarin has been the single most effective treatment to prevent stroke in AF patients, representing the mainstay of OAC. Warfarin exerts its anticoagulant effect by interfering with the biosyntheses of coagulation factors in the liver. Vitamin K acts as an essential cofactor for a specific carboxylation reaction that converts clotting factors into biologically active forms. Thus by inhibiting this carboxylation process warfarin leads to the synthesis of ineffective coagulants.

Warfarin was initially compared to placebo or control in several trials of stroke prevention in AF, and has justifiably been part of standard recommendations (Laupacis et al. 1992; Matchar et al. 1994). These trials included over 4000 patients with non-valvular

Table 6.3 HAS-BLED score for the assessment of the bleeding risk		
Letter	Clinical characteristics	Points assigned
H	Hypertension, i.e. uncontrolled blood pressure	1
A	Abnormal renal and liver function	1 or 2
S	Stroke	1
B	Bleeding tendency or predisposition	1
L	Labile INRs	1
E	Elderly (age > 65 years, frail condition)	1
D	Drugs or alcohol	1 or 2
		Maximum 9 points

or no rheumatic AF, and demonstrated that anticoagulation with adjusted-dose warfarin was superior to aspirin or placebo as far as stroke risk in AF patients is concerned. Overall, adjusted-dose warfarin reduces the risk of stroke by 64% and mortality by 26% compared to placebo (Hart et al. 2007, 2009). The relative risk reduction compared to aspirin was about 50%. Warfarin was effective in all age groups and in both men and women. In addition, warfarin provides significant benefit in patients who have already had a stroke.

In the Atrial fibrillation Clopidogrel Trial with Irbesartan for prevention of Vascular Events–Warfarin arm (ACTIVE W) trial (ACTIVE Writing Group of the ACTIVE Investigators et al. 2006), anticoagulation therapy was superior to the combination of clopidogrel plus aspirin with no difference in bleeding events between treatment arms.

The ACTIVE A trial (Connolly et al. 2009b) found that although the combination of aspirin and clopidogrel was superior to aspirin monotherapy in reducing major vascular events in AF patients (by 28%, primarily driven by the reduction in the rate of stroke), although combination therapy to increased rates of major bleeding (approximately 2%). Thus, aspirin in combination with clopidogrel could be considered in AF patients when warfarin is unsuitable or where patients refuse to receive warfarin, but not as an alternative to VKA in patients at high bleeding risk.

Despite being highly effective, warfarin has several limitations and drawbacks that have led to its underuse in clinical practice (Bungard et al. 2000). One study that included 3600 patients with AF or atrial flutter in a community database (2000 to 2007) concluded that only 53% of patients received anticoagulation therapy as recommended by current guidelines (Gorin et al. 2010). Indeed, warfarin has a narrow therapeutic window and requires careful laboratory monitoring and clinical follow up in order to maintain the INR in the target therapeutic range. This need for anticoagulation monitoring represents a considerable inconvenience, especially in remote dwelling AF patients. In addition to that, major bleeding occurs in 1–3% of AF patients receiving warfarin per year. Furthermore, warfarin has a slow onset and offset of action. Indeed, effective levels of anticoagulation are obtained only after several days of warfarin use, and its anticoagulant effect reduces slowly after interruption.

Additionally, warfarin demonstrates considerable variability in dose and metabolism within and between patients and it is subject to multiple food and drug interactions. Another complicating factor is that proteins C and S, which are endogenous anticoagulants, are also inhibited by warfarin. Taking into consideration that protein C has a short half-life of only 8 hours, compared to the long half-lives of some vitamin K-dependent coagulation factors, warfarin therapy may also produce a hypercoagulable state until the full effect of warfarin is achieved. Thus, overlap with heparin is required for 3–5 days in order to protect patients from thrombotic complications.

Given the many reasons that contributed to the underuse of warfarin in patients with AF, warfarin is often not used and even when it is, rates of discontinuation are high (Birman-Deych et al. 2006; Hylek et al. 2007). Furthermore, many patients receiving warfarin still have inadequate or suboptimal quality of anticoagulation (Connolly et al. 2008).

Recent surveys suggest that the use of warfarin have reached a plateau in the past few years at approximately 50–60% of eligible patients with AF (Go et al. 1999; Waldo et al. 2005; Birman-Deych et al. 2006; Nieuwlatt et al. 2006; Hylek et al. 2007). Thus, a high percentage of AF patients are either unprotected against stroke or undertreated with antiplatelets. The unmet clinical needs owing to the pharmacological limitations of warfarin led to the development of new anticoagulants that not only display favourable pharmacological profile but also to be effective, safe, and convenient to use.

The characteristics of the ideal anticoagulant agent for AF might include the following:

- High degree of protection against stroke or embolism.
- Wide therapeutic window, low risk of bleeding.
- A rapid onset and offset of action.
- Oral administration.
- Low binding with plasma proteins.
- A predictable antithrombotic response.
- Freedom from drug and food interactions.
- Low incidence of significant adverse effects.
- No need for routine monitoring reversibility of anticoagulant effect.
- Relatively low cost.

6.5 **New anticoagulant agents**

New OAC drugs are emerging as alternatives to warfarin for the prevention of thrombotic complications in patients with non-valvular AF. The aim was to produce medications which fulfil the conditions for the ideal anticoagulant. Novel anticoagulant agents are low-molecular-weight synthetic molecules that inhibit the activity of one single step in the coagulation cascade.

New oral anticoagulant agents (NOACs) are classified in two main categories: (1) the oral direct thrombin inhibitors (e.g. dabigatran) and (2) the oral direct factor Xa inhibitors (e.g. rivaroxaban, apixaban, etc.).

6.5.1 **Dabigatran etexilate**

Dabigatran etexilate is the prodrug of dabigatran, a potent, non-peptidic synthetic molecule that specifically and reversibly inhibits both free and clot-bound thrombin (Hauel et al. 2002; van Ryn et al. 2007; Wienen et al. 2007). Currently guidelines suggest that dabigatran can be considered as an alternative to warfarin in patients with non-valvular, paroxysmal or permanent AF with risk factors for stroke or systemic embolism (Camm et al. 2012).

Dabigatran etexilate is converted by a serum esterase to the active compound (dabigatran) in the liver. The onset of action of dabigatran is fast with peak plasma concentrations and maximal anticoagulant effects achieved within 0.5–4 hours. The half-life is 17 hours with multiple doses (Stangier et al. 2007) and the basic route of elimination is via the kidneys (Stangier et al. 2007). In patients with moderate (creatinine clearance (CrCl) 30–49 mL/min) or severe renal impairment (CrCl < 30 mL/min) dabigatran may exhibit prolonged excretion rates (Stangier et al. 2010; European Medicines Agency n.d.). Thus, dabigatran is not recommended in patients with severe renal dysfunction (CrCl < 30 mL/min) (Camm et al. 2012).

Assessment of renal function (by CrCl) using the Cockcroft–Gault formula is mandatory prior to starting treatment with dabigatran. Renal function should be also assessed annually in patients with normal (CrCl ≥ 80 mL/min) or mild (CrCl 50–79 mL/min) renal decline, and perhaps two to three times per year in patients with moderate (i.e. creatinine clearance 30–49 mL/min) renal decline.

Oral administration of dabigatran etexilate delivers predictable and favourable pharmacokinetic and pharmacodynamic effects and does not require routine coagulation monitoring or dose adjustment. In addition to that it is associated with few known drug interactions.

In general, dabigatran etexilate is also well tolerated, although it is associated with a higher rate of dyspepsia than warfarin.

Dabigatran displays low (35%) plasma protein binding, implying that displacement interactions are unlikely to affect its pharmacokinetics and pharmacodynamics (Blech et al. 2008). Food intake affects the time to peak plasma dabigatran levels without affecting overall bioavailability (Stangier et al. 2005).

Based on the results of the RE-LY (Randomized Evaluation of Long-term anticoagulant therapy with dabigatran etexilate) trial (Connolly et al. 2009a, 2010), dabigatran etexilate has been approved by both the Food and Drug Administration (FDA) and the European Medicines Agency (EMA), as well as in many countries worldwide, for prevention of thromboembolic complications in patients with non-valvular AF with at least one additional risk factor (previous stroke, TIA, or systemic embolism; left ventricular ejection fraction (LVEF) < 40%; symptomatic heart failure; and age $\geq$ 75 years or age $\geq$ 65 years with one of the following: diabetes, coronary artery disease, or hypertension). The FDA has approved the 150 mg twice daily dose, and the 75 mg twice daily dose in patients with severe renal impairment (CrCl 15–30 mL/min). On the other hand, the EMA has approved the 150 mg twice-daily and 110 mg twice-daily doses.

The RE-LY trial was a large randomized controlled trial of over 18,000 patients from 951 centres in 44 countries comparing the efficacy and safety of dabigatran with warfarin for prevention of stroke or systemic thromboembolism in patients with non-valvular AF and at least one additional risk factor for stroke were enrolled. The RE-LY trial found that dabigatran administered at a dose of 110 mg twice daily was associated with rates of stroke and systemic embolism that were similar to those associated with warfarin, as well as 20% lower rates of major haemorrhage (defined as a reduction in haemoglobin level of 2 g/dL, bleeding requiring transfusion requiring at least 2 units of blood, or symptomatic bleeding in a critical area or organ). Dabigatran administered at a dose of 150 mg twice daily was superior to warfarin in regard to reduction in stroke or systemic embolism but had similar rates of major haemorrhage (Connolly et al. 2009a).

Apart from renal function, caution is required in elderly patients (older than 80) and in patients who receive potent P-glycoprotein (P-gp) inhibitors (azole-antimycotics, immunosuppressants, and human immunodeficiency virus protease inhibitors must be avoided), or P-gp inducers (potent P-gp inducers such us rifampicin are also contraindicated). Given that verapamil which is also a P-gp inhibitor may increase plasma concentrations of dabigatran, its concomitant use require a dose reduction. As far as amiodarone and quinidine are concerned, no dose adjustment is required. On the other hand, dronedarone is a potent inhibitor of P-gp efflux transporter and should be avoided in patients receiving dabigatran because it may lead to increased dabigatran plasma levels.

Concurrent treatment with non-steroidal anti-inflammatory drugs (NSAIDs) significantly increases the risk of major bleeding and requires a careful benefit–risk assessment. Dabigatran should only be given if the benefit outweighs the risk of bleeding. Concomitant treatment with any other anticoagulants is contraindicated except in case of switching therapy to or from dabigatran or when *unfractionated* heparin (UFH) is administered at doses necessary to maintain the patency of central venous or arterial catheters.

Synoptically, the 110 mg twice daily dose is recommended for:

- Elderly, that is, age > 80 years.
- CrCl 30–50 mL/min and a high risk of bleeding, including age 75–80 years.
- Concomitant use of P-gp inducers or inhibitors.
- High bleeding risk (HAS-BLED $\geq$ 3)

A secondary finding from the RE-LY trial was a numerical but non-significant increase in the rate of MI when compared with warfarin. A recent meta-analysis of randomized trials comparing oral direct thrombin inhibitors with warfarin for stroke prevention in AF revealed significantly higher MI rates in the dabigatran and combined ximelagatran and dabigatran group, which the authors suggested as a possible direct thrombin inhibitor class-specific effect (Artang et al. 2012). However, meta-analysis of warfarin versus other treatments demonstrated a lower MI rate with warfarin (Lip and Lane 2010), and reflect that warfarin has protective effects against MI. Thus, the difference regarding the rate of MI could be attributed to the fact that dabigatran simply is not protective against MI as well as warfarin.

6.5.2 Rivaroxaban

The oral factor Xa inhibitor, rivaroxaban, is another NOAC that has been expected to revolutionize stroke prevention in AF patients. Notably rivaroxaban remains the only FDA-approved anticoagulant that offers once-daily dosing without the need for routine blood monitoring (Fleming et al. 2011).

Based on the 14,000-participant Rivaroxaban Once Daily Oral Direct Factor Xa Inhibition Compared with Vitamin K Antagonism for Prevention of Stroke and Embolism Trial in Atrial Fibrillation (ROCKET AF) it was the second of the three drugs to receive FDA approval in November of 2011. The ROCKET AF trial (Patel 2011) determined that rivaroxaban is non-inferior to warfarin for the prevention of stroke or systemic embolism. The trial also revealed that there was no difference in the risk of major bleeding, although fatal and intracranial bleeding occurred less frequently in the rivaroxaban group. In addition, a not significant reduction in MI was observed in patients receiving rivaroxaban compared to placebo.

Rivaroxaban is a competitive reversible inhibitor of activated factor X (Xa) which is the active component of the prothrombinase complex that catalyses transformation of prothrombin (factor II) to thrombin (factor IIa). The drug is a small molecule with a bioavailability of 80% and peak plasma concentrations occurring 2.5 to 4 hours after oral administration. The rivaroxaban dose should be administrated after food since absorption rate and bioavailability are reduced in fasted patients.

The half-life of rivaroxaban is 5–13 hours. Approximately 50% of rivaroxaban is metabolized by liver enzymes. There are no known active metabolites. Rivaroxaban has a dual mechanism of excretion. Approximately 66% of the dose is excreted via the kidneys and the remainder is eliminated by the faecal–biliary route. Because of a high degree of albumin binding in plasma (92–95%), rivaroxaban is not dialysable. Thus rivaroxaban anticoagulation effects are not reversed by haemodialysis.

The recommended dose for AF patients with normal renal function is 20 mg once daily. Even though rivaroxaban is less dependent on renal elimination the recommended dose in patients with moderate renal impairment (CrCl 30–49 mL/min) is 15 mg once daily. In the European Society of Cardiology (ESC) guidelines, the use of rivaroxaban is not recommended in patients with a severe renal impairment (CrCl < 30 mL/min) (Camm et al. 2012). Furthermore, rivaroxaban should be avoided in patients with moderate–severe hepatic impairment (Food and Drug Administration 2013). In patients with mild hepatic impairment no dose adjustment is required. Rivaroxaban is also contraindicated during pregnancy.

Concomitant use of combined P-gp and cytochrome (CYP)-3A4 strong inhibitors and inducers must be avoided owing to the fact that they may increase or reduce, respectively, plasma levels of rivaroxaban. Similar to dabigatran rivaroxaban has favourable pharmacokinetic and pharmacodynamic characteristics that render unnecessary routine coagulation monitoring. In addition few drug–drug interactions between rivaroxaban and common medications have been found.

Rivaroxaban (similar to dabigatran etexilate and apixaban) is a substrate of P-gp. Concomitant use of drugs which are strong inhibitors of CYP-3A4 or P-gp efflux transporter (e.g. systemic ketoconazole, itraconazole) leading to increased rivaroxaban anti-coagulant effect. Thus, the concomitant use of these drugs should be avoided. Moreover, potent inducers of CYP-3A4 and/or P-gp efflux transporter should be avoided due to the significant decrease in rivaroxaban plasma levels.

In addition, concomitant use of NSAIDs and platelet aggregation inhibitors should be undertaken with caution due to increased bleeding risk. Due to the increased haemorrhagic risk, concurrent treatment with other antithrombotic drugs is contraindicated. However, UFH may be administered at doses necessary to maintain an open central venous or arterial catheter or in case of switching therapy to or from rivaroxaban. In general, rivaroxaban is otherwise well tolerated. The most common adverse event associated with the use of rivaroxaban is bleeding.

6.5.3 **Apixaban**

Apixaban which is an inhibitor of the active site of factor Xa, was approved by European Commission and FDA for the prevention of stroke or systemic embolism in patients with non-valvular AF-based on the findings of the ARISTOTLE (Granger et al. 2011) and AVERROES trials (Connolly et al. 2011).

The ARISTOTLE trial demonstrated that treatment with apixaban led to significant reduction in stroke or systemic embolism and mortality. The use of apixaban also resulted in lower rates of major bleeding and of intracranial bleeding. In addition, patients receiving apixaban had a lower rate of MI than those on warfarin.

On the other hand, the AVERROES trial assessed apixaban in relation to aspirin for the prevention of stroke in patients who were at high risk of stroke but unsuitable for VKA therapy. Apixaban was found to be superior to aspirin in both efficacy and safety.

Apixaban is a small molecule which is rapidly absorbed, with a bioavailability of 50%. Peak plasma concentrations are achieved within 3 to 4 hours after oral administration and its half-life is approximately 12 hours (Raghavan et al. 2009). Apixaban may be admin-istered without regard to food intake. Apixaban is metabolized in the liver mainly by CYP-3A4 and to some extent via CYP-independent pathways into inactive metabolites (Raghavan et al. 2009). Apixaban does not inhibit or induce CYP enzymes and thus, the potential of drug interaction is significantly reduced. However, co-administration of drugs that are substrates for inducers or inhibitors of CYP-3A4 may significantly affect its plasma levels. Additionally, strong inhibitors of both CYP-3A4 and P-gp should be avoided due to increased plasma concentrations of apixaban. Particular caution is also required in case of concomitant use of strong inducers of both CYP-3A4 and P-gp that may lead to reduced plasma apixaban levels.

Particular caution is required if patients receive concomitantly drugs which affect haemo-stasis such as NSAID, acetylsalicylic acid (ASA), and other antiplatelet drugs. Concurrent treatment with any other anticoagulants is contraindicated except when converting patients to or from apixaban or when UFH is administrated in order to maintain a patent central venous or arterial catheter.

Similarly to rivaroxaban, apixaban exhibits a dual mechanism of excretion. Approximately 25% is eliminated via the kidneys, whereas the remainder is excreted in the faeces. Owing to high level of protein binding (~87%) is not dialysable. Thus apixaban anticoagulation effects are not reversed through haemodialysis.

Table 6.4 Comparison of pharmacokinetic and pharmacodynamic characteristics of three new oral anticoagulants

	Apixaban	Rivaroxaban	Dabigatran
Bioavailability	50%	60–80%	6%
C_{max}	3 hours	3 hours	3 hours
Half-life	9–14 hours	5–13 hours	12–17 hours
Elimination	27% renal 73% hepatic	33% renal active 33% renal inactive 33% hepatic	80% renal 20% hepatic
Dose	5 mg twice daily	20 mg once daily	150 mg twice daily/110 mg twice daily
Monitoring	No	No	No
Interactions	CYP3A4 P-gp	CYP3A4 P-gp	P-gp

The recommended dose for AF patients is 5 mg twice daily in patients with non-valvular AF. Mild to moderate impairment of renal function does not significantly affect anti-factor Xa activity of apixaban and thus in the United States and Canada, no dosage amendment is recommended in patients with isolated mild to moderate renal dysfunction. This is particularly important if we take into account that approximately 20% of patients with AF also have some renal dysfunction (Marinigh et al. 2011).

Notwithstanding, the apixaban dose should be reduced to 2.5 mg twice daily in patients with two of the following three criteria: serum creatinine of at least 1.5 mg/dL, age 80 years or over, or body weight of 60 kg or lower. Even though apixaban is less affected by renal dysfunction than dabigatran, in individuals with severe renal impairment (CrCl 15–29 mL/min), apixaban plasma concentrations were significantly increased, exposing patients to high bleeding risk. Thus, the use of apixaban in patients with creatinine clearance lower than 25–30 mL/min, or in patients undergoing dialysis, it is not recommended in the ESC guidelines. Apixaban is also contraindicated in the case of severe hepatic impairment. Hypersensitivity to the active substance or to any of the excipients represents additional contraindication to receiving apixaban

The pharmacokinetic and pharmacodynamic characteristics of the novel oral anticoagulants are depicted in Table 6.4.

Despite promising trial results and updated guidelines for the prevention of AF-related stroke or systemic embolism, novel drugs have some difficulties and potential limitations.

Indeed, some of the favourable characteristics advantages of the NOAC agents might turn out to be important drawbacks in certain clinical scenarios (Box 6.1). In particular, the absence of routine laboratory monitoring leads to the physician's inability to assess patient compliance. Additionally, coagulation testing, although cumbersome in most cases, may also be helpful in the context of bleeding.

Similarly, fast onset and offset of the novel anticoagulants in comparison with warfarin could represent a drawback in these patients owing to the fact that omission of one single dose might lead to hypercoagulability and increased risk of stroke. Another important disadvantage of the NOACs is the lack of specifics antidotes able to reverse anticoagulant effects of NOACs. Furthermore, dabigatran and apixaban require twice-daily dosing, which

Box 6.1 Summary of potential limitations of new anticoagulants

- No known specific antidote (yet)
- Absence of well established tests to monitor anticoagulant effect
- Long-term safety profile is not established
- Preoperative management of patients on NOACs is not well consolidated
- Cost-effectiveness compared to warfarin is remained to be clarified in patients with very well controlled INR
- Absence of head-to-head trials of new agents
- Dabigatran and apixaban are given twice daily
- Dyspepsia is a commonly reported side effect with dabigatran

could potentially associated to reduced patient compliance a consequently to decreased efficacy of the treatment.

Another key concept related to NOACs is the fact that there is relatively limited evidence regarding their long-term use. Taking into consideration that AF patients usually require life-long treatment, the limited clinical experience with long-term use of NOACs represent an important restrictive factor in relation to their adoption in everyday clinical practice.

In order to bridge the gap of evidence related to the long-term use of dabigatran, the RELY-ABLE Study (Connolly et al. 2013) has provided additional support to the safety profile and efficacy of dabigatran for stroke prevention in patients with non-valvular AF over a period of 2.3 years of follow up. The new long-term results are concordant with the results derived from the landmark RE-LY trial. In particular, RELY-ABLE confirmed that dabigatran 150 mg was superior to 110 mg for stroke prevention, at the cost of slightly increased risk of bleeding complications. The rate of major bleedings including intracranial haemorrhage appeared to be slightly more common in the RELY-ABLE trial than in RE-LY, but still at a low rate. Moreover, dabigatran 110 mg was associated with a significantly lower risk of major bleeding and a trend toward reduced risk of intracranial haemorrhage compared with dabigatran 150 mg. No difference was found in the rates of gastrointestinal (GI) bleeding between both doses in RELY-ABLE.

The safety of the treatment with apixaban is currently being studied in the long-term, open-label extension phase of the AVERROES study (LTOLE). As far as rivaroxaban is concerned there is a lack of long-term safety data and its safety has not been specifically demonstrated in people at high risk of bleeding.

After the approval of NOACs for patients with non-valvular AF, great concern was raised about the matter of cost. On the other hand, patients with severe renal impairment, severe liver disease, patients who are pregnant or breastfeeding, patients unable to afford the cost of NOACs, and patients predicted to receive interacting medications are not considered good candidates for the NOACs. There have been some data addressing the issue of the cost-effectiveness of NOACs. Except for patients with optimal control of INR, both dabigatran and rivaroxaban appear to be a cost-effective alternative to adjusted-dose warfarin for stroke prevention in AF (Freeman et al. 2011; Pink et al. 2011; Shah and Gage 2011; Sorensen et al. 2011; Lee et al. 2012). In a recent study carried out in Canada, an indirect treatment comparison of dabigatran versus rivaroxaban was performed which suggested that dabigatran was associated with a lower risk of intracranial haemorrhage, and was superior to rivaroxaban in regard to acute care and long-term follow-up costs per patient which compensated for the difference in drug costs (Kansal et al. 2012).

In addition, in RE-LY and in the ROCKET-AF study, both doses of dabigatran and rivaroxaban 20 mg once daily respectively, showed a significantly higher rate of GI bleeds compared to warfarin. Currently there is no evidence that support that apixaban is associated with increased risk of GI bleeding. In fact in ARISTOTLE study the incidence of GI bleeds was lower with apixaban compared to warfarin.

Thus, before initiating NOACs it is of crucial importance that all factors known to increase the risk of GI bleeding should be recognized. Elderly patients, patients with a history of GI bleeding or patients with GI tract pathology, could be at increased of GI bleeding. In addition, their use should be avoided in patients with active peptic ulcer disease or history of recent GI bleeding.

A recent study that assessed the efficacy and safety of dabigatran in an 'everyday clinical practice' population revealed that despite the fact that there was no difference in major bleeding risk between dabigatran (both doses) and warfarin, GI bleeding was lower with dabigatran 110 mg (adjusted hazard ratio: 0.60, 95% confidence interval: 0.37–0.93) compared to warfarin (Larsen et al. 2013). Thus, patients at high risk of bleeding taking dabigatran could be considered for the lower daily dose (110 mg twice daily).

Additionally, a recent study in the United States used reviewed data from the RE-LY, ROCKET-AF, and ARISTOTLE trials in order to calculate the medical cost savings associated with the use of NOACs. In this study, use of dabigatran, rivaroxaban, and apixaban was associated with annual savings of US$179, US$89, and US$485 per patient-year, respectively, compared with warfarin (Deitelzweig et al. 2012). These promising results are mainly related to the cost of major bleeding events, hospital admissions, or emergency department visits for out-of-range INRs, not to the drug costs themselves, which may reach US$3000 per year for any of the NOACs (compared with a modest US$48 per year for warfarin).

Consequently, good candidates for the NOACs are patients with the following characteristics:

- Contraindication to warfarin but not an NOAC.
- Patients who are not likely to receive drugs that interact with NOACs.
- Patients that are not able to achieve a INR time in therapeutic range (TTR) with warfarin of at least 65%.
- Patients with known excess use of ethanol.
- Patients who are predicted to have significant difficulties with INR monitoring.
- CrCl greater than 30mL/min.
- Patients who have a very high risk of stroke may derive benefit from the rapid anticoagulation offered by NOACs.
- No history of coagulopathy related to liver disease.
- Patients with high bleeding risk assessed by HAS-BLED score where dabigatran 110 mg twice-daily dosing should be considered.

NOACs could also represent the first choice in elderly patients given that they were superior to warfarin in relation to both stroke prevention and major bleeding, including intracranial haemorrhage compared with warfarin. This represents an important advantage of NOACs since 45% of the patients diagnosed with AF are older than 75 years (Go et al. 2001).

With the emergence of the NOACs, one challenge is to perhaps identify those patients who could potentially do well on a VKA, with a high TTR. The SAMe-TT$_2$R$_2$ score (Table 6.5) could have an important role here, by predicting those who could do well on warfarin

| Table 6.5 The SAMe-TT$_2$R$_2$ score for predicting patients that would do well on VKAs, with high time in therapeutic range |||
Acronym	Definitions	Points
S	Sex (female)	1
A	Age (less than 60 years)	1
M	Medical history[a]	1
e		
T	Treatment (interacting treatment, e.g. amiodarone for rhythm control)	1
T	Tobacco use (within 2 years)	2
R	Race (non-Caucasian)	2 Maximum 8 points

[a]Two of the following: hypertension, diabetes, myocardial infarction, peripheral artery disease, congestive heart failure, previous stroke, pulmonary disease, hepatic or renal disease.

(SAMe-TT$_2$R$_2$ score 0–1) or those who are likely to have poor anticoagulation control if warfarin is used (SAMe-TT$_2$R$_2$ score ≥ 2) where a NOAC could represent a better option (Apostolakis et al. 2013) (Table 6.5).

Overall, NOACs which can be easily managed without the need for routine monitoring represent a reliable alternative to warfarin in the setting of the management of newly diagnosed AF patients at high risk of stroke. Notably, a recent analysis revealed that the three NOACs had an edge on warfarin in patients with AF at high risk of stroke regardless of the bleeding risk.

In addition, excluding patients with a CHA$_2$DS$_2$-VASc of 0, almost all patients with AF treatment with NOACs were associated with net clinical benefit compared to treatment with warfarin regardless of HASBLED score. Interestingly patients with higher HAS-BLED score were more likely to benefit from NOACs (Olesen et al. 2011; Friberg et al. 2012).

Although NOACs have demonstrated their efficacy safety profile by being separately compared to warfarin in large clinical trials, there is no evidence to support the recommendation for or against any of the NOACs over each other. Large-scale head-to-head randomized studies which support one agent over the other are not yet available. Indirect comparisons of the NOACs have been published, although this method is associated with certain limitations which are mainly related to the differences in the pharmacological properties, the study designs, and the heterogeneity of the populations studied.

In a recent indirect comparison study of the three NOACs, there was no profound significant differences in efficacy between apixaban and dabigatran etexilate (both doses) or rivaroxaban (Lip et al. 2012). With regard to major bleeding, apixaban and dabigatran 110 mg twice daily were safer than dabigatran 150 mg twice daily and rivaroxaban. On the other hand, dabigatran 150 mg twice daily was superior to rivaroxaban for some efficacy endpoints, whereas major bleeding was significantly lower with dabigatran 110 mg twice daily or apixaban.

Another indirect comparison study that focused on the secondary prevention subgroups of all three trials found there was no difference among apixaban, dabigatran, and rivaroxaban with regard to efficacy for the main endpoints. The stroke rate in the primary prevention cohort was considerably less common with dabigatran 150 mg twice daily compared with apixaban but at the cost of increased major bleeding and GI bleeding events. Dabigatran 110 mg twice daily compared with rivaroxaban was associated with lower rates of haemorrhagic stroke, vascular death, major bleeding, and intracranial bleeding but with higher rates of MI events. Apixaban compared with rivaroxaban did not differ as far as the efficacy is concerned but major bleeding was more common with rivaroxaban than with apixaban. No significant differences for safety and efficacy were found between dabigatran 150 mg twice daily and rivaroxaban (Rasmussen et al. 2012). Similar observations have been reported in other studies (Mantha and Ansell 2012).

Notwithstanding, there are certain clinical circumstances in which a specific anticoagulant agent is preferred over the other. This fact is related to the risk–benefit profile of NOACs and the patient's characteristics. Thus, it is now considered that one size does not fit all, and we can fit the drug to the individual patient's characteristics.

Thus, a more efficacious and less safe agent may better suit patients at a very high risk for stroke and a low risk of bleeding while a less effective but safer agent would be more suitable for patients with a moderate stroke risk but a high bleeding risk.

Dabigatran is the only novel anticoagulant agent that could be used in two different, evidence-based dosing schemes. This represents an important asset given that it provides the possibility of dosing adjustment of dabigatran in order to meet the individual clinical needs. Apart from that, there are also data on dabigatran that support its use as a valid alternative to warfarin in the setting of elective cardioversion.

On the other hand, in patients presenting with GI upset or dyspepsia related to dabigatran it is recommended the substitution of the later with another NOAC agent.

Furthermore, given that only 25% of apixaban is excreted via the kidneys and taking into account the promising results of apixaban in patients with moderate renal impairment, it could be inferred that apixaban has an edge over the other agents in this setting. The patient's preferences may also be a consideration, for example, some patients might prefer rivaroxaban because of its advantage of once-daily administration. In fact this factor appears to be important since it may be related to the enhancement of patient's compliance.

6.6 Specific coagulation tests—antidotes, reversal strategies

A worthwhile practical consideration regarding the use of NOACs in clinical practice is the absence of specific coagulation tests that are able to assess the anticoagulation intensity attributed to NOACs. The INR is not appropriate for the qualitative assessment of the anticoagulant effects of NOACs and should therefore not be used in this setting.

In the case of dabigatran there are simple coagulation tests such us the ecarin clotting time (ECT) and thrombin clotting time (TCT) that are sensitive tests in order to check the presence of anticoagulation effects of dabigatran (van Ryn et al. 2010). A normal TCT or ECT rules out the presence of important levels of dabigatran. Nevertheless, these tests simply tell of an anticoagulation effect, and not anticoagulation intensity, and are not specific for drug dose adjustments.

For example, the activated partial thromboplastin time (aPTT) is also useful in order to obtain qualitative measure of anticoagulation status, attributed to dabigatran, especially in the context of surgical emergencies. In this context a normal aPTT result will indicate a lack of residual anticoagulant effect. There is no linear correlation between the anticoagulation intensity attributed to dabigatran and aPTT (van Ryn et al. 2010; Huisman et al. 2012).

The prothrombin time (PT) is also useful as a qualitative indicator of the presence of rivaroxaban but is not related to the anticoagulant effect of rivaroxaban. Thus, a normal aPTT or PT in the setting of dabigatran or rivaroxaban, respectively, would suggest that haemostatic function is not impaired because of the drug.

Although apixaban at therapeutic levels is expected to prolong PT, INR, and aPTT, these coagulation tests should be not used to assess the anticoagulant effects of apixaban. Notably, the anti-Xa assay provides a more reliable quantitative assessment of the anticoagulant effect for the oral factor Xa inhibitors (Barrett et al. 2010; Tripodi et al. 2011). Indeed, the Xa assay has been proved to be sensitive to lower amounts of rivaroxaban and apixaban with less variability and may help evaluate the direct effects of these novel agents. Indeed, chromogenic-based anti-Xa assays are currently considered reasonably sensitive screening tests for the presence of rivaroxaban and apixaban (Samama and Guinet 2011; Eby 2013).

The calibrated Hemoclot Thrombin Inhibitor assay, although not sufficiently studied, represents a promising coagulant test in the setting of laboratory assessment of anticoagulation activity attributed to dabigatran (van Ryn et al. 2010; Huisman et al. 2012; Stangier and Feuring 2012). In particular, this test is considered more sensitive and appropriate for assessing anticoagulant effects of dabigatran in relation to the other coagulation tests. In particular, the Hemoclot Thrombin Inhibitor assay is a sensitive diluted thrombin time assay which exhibits a direct linear correlation between dabigatran levels and clotting (van Ryn et al. 2010).

6.6.1 **Management of bleeding**

One important shortcoming of the NOACs is that they have neither specific antidote nor well-established procedures of reversal of their anticoagulants effects. This is particularly important because anticoagulation always carries a risk of haemorrhagic complications. Thus the management of bleeding complications consists primarily in supportive measures rather than administration of specific antidotes. Based on the ESC guidelines, the assessment of haemodynamic condition and the use of coagulation assays is initially recommended in order to starkly assess the anticoagulation status (aPTT for dabigatran, PT or anti-Xa activity for rivaroxaban) and the assessment of renal and liver function. Subsequent management is individualized according to the severity of haemorrhage.

In cases of minor haemorrhage it is essential that the next dose be postponed or omitted. In fact, given the short half-life of NOACs, their plasma levels are expected to decline rapidly. In addition to that, since dabigatran has mainly renal excretion, maintenance of adequate dieresis is important. In cases of bleeding attributed to the anticoagulant effects of dabigatran, haemodialysis and should be also considered. Indeed dabigatran is dialysable due to its relative low plasma protein binding.

In cases of moderate severe bleeding or in cases of minor haemorrhage in which previous measures turn out to be ineffective apart of supportive strategies to control bleeding, mechanical compression, fluid administration, transfusion of blood products, and oral charcoal are considered very important. In the event of very severe bleeding or when all previous measures failed to control bleeding efficiently, non-specific reversal agents such as recombinant activated factor VII or prothrombin complex concentrate have been proposed in order to reverse the effects of NOACs. However, further research is also needed in order to elucidate the role of recombinant-activated factor VIIa in the management of bleeding complications in patients receiving NOACs (Warkentin et al. 2012).

Fresh frozen plasma (FFP) does not reverse the anticoagulant effect of NOACs and thus its use as a reversal agent is not expected to be useful. However, FFP could be useful as plasma expander during acute bleeding (Heidbuchel et al. 2013). A phase 2 study evaluating the efficacy safety profile of a new investigational universal antidote for Factor Xa inhibitor anticoagulants (PRT4445) has recently commenced. PRT4445 is a novel recombinant protein aiming to reverse the anticoagulant effects of Factor Xa inhibitors in certain clinical situation as in case of major bleeding. Notably, PRT4445 has already been evaluated in preclinical studies which provided evidence supporting its safety, efficacy in reversing the anticoagulant effects of all Factor Xa inhibitors (Hutchaleelaha et al. 2012; Lu et al. 2013).

6.7 **Perioperative management**

Currently there is also limited evidence with the perioperative management of patients on NOACs. Particular caution is required in patients with therapeutic levels of drugs since, unlike warfarin, prolonged bleeding times cannot be reversed. Given the short half-lives of NOACs in patients with normal renal function, the interruption for at least 24–48 hours or at least 2–3 days when renal function is impaired (CrCl is < 50 mL/min) should be sufficient to ensure adequate haemostasis prior to invasive or surgical procedures. Thus, perioperative management should be individualized taking in considerations four parameters:

- The bleeding risk.
- The risk of thrombosis.
- The type of surgery planned.
- The renal function of the patient.

In cases of patients who undergo intervention with no clinically important haemorrhagic risk such as cataract, glaucoma, or dental procedures it is recommended that the intervention is planned for 18–24 hours after the last intake of the anticoagulant. Notwithstanding, performing these interventions 12 or 24 hours after the last intake, based on twice- or once-daily dosing may represent a reasonable strategy, especially in cases of patients at high risk of thromboembolic events (Heidbuchel et al. 2013).

In patients with normal renal function who are at standard risk of bleeding it is suggested to discontinue NOACs for 24 hours before elective surgical procedures (Flaker et al. 2012). In cases of patients undergoing procedures that carry a high risk of major haemorrhagic complications, it is recommended to stop NOACs 48 hours in advance, provided that they have normal renal function. If the risk of bleeding is high, a normal aPTT or PT result in the setting of dabigatran or rivaroxaban, respectively, would suggest a lack of residual anticoagulant effect (van Ryn et al. 2010; Samama and Guinet 2011).

In patients with high thrombotic risk who undergo intervention associated with minor bleeding risk, treatment with NOACs should be maintained without interruption. Notably, the period of discontinuation increases with decreasing renal function. Indeed, especially for dabigatran, half-life is protracted in cases of renal impairment.

In patients taking dabigatran who undergo low bleeding risk procedures the last dabigatran dose should be administrated 36 hours before surgery in patients with mildly impaired renal function (CrCl 50–80 mL/min) and 48 hours before surgery in patients with moderate impaired renal function (CrCl 30–50mL/min). In cases of patients with renal dysfunction that are scheduled to undergo high bleeding risk procedures, the period of discontinuation of dabigatran should be longer. As described in Table 6.6, in patients with mild and moderate renal impairment dabigatran should be interrupted at least 72 hours and 96 hours respectively prior to the procedure.

In patients taking rivaroxaban or apixaban, preoperative drug interruption depends on the drug elimination half-life, the renal function, and the drug dependence on renal excretion (33% for rivaroxaban, 25% for apixaban). As shown in Table 6.6, it is recommended that both rivaroxaban and apixaban should be discontinued at least 24 hours before low bleeding risk procedures. Notwithstanding, in patients with severe renal impairment (CrCl 15–30 mL/min) the period of interruption of both rivaroxaban and apixaban should be

Table 6.6 A suggested management approach for perioperative cessation of NOACs

	Low bleeding risk procedures	High bleeding risk procedures
Dabigatran CrCl > 80 mL/min CrCl 50–80 mL/min CrCl 30–50 mL/min CrCl 15–30 mL/min CrCl < 15 mL/min	Last dose: ≥ 24 hours Last dose: ≥ 36hours Last dose: ≥ 48hours Not indicated No official indication for use	Last dose ≥ 48 hours Last dose: ≥ 72 hours Last dose: ≥ 96 hours Not indicated No official indication for use
Rivaroxaban CrCl > 80 mL/min CrCl 50–80 mL/min CrCl 30–50 mL/min CrCl 15–30 mL/min CrCl < 15 mL/min	Last dose: ≥ 24 hours Last dose: ≥ 24hours Last dose: ≥ 24hours Last dose: ≥ 36hours No official indication for use	Last dose: ≥ 48 hours Last dose: ≥ 48 hours Last dose: ≥ 48 hours Last dose: ≥ 48 hours No official indication for use
Apixaban CrCl > 80 mL/min CrCl 50–80 mL/min CrCl 30–50 mL/min CrCl 15–30 mL/min CrCl < 15 mL/min	Last dose: ≥ 24 hours Last dose: ≥ 24hours Last dose: ≥ 24hours Last dose: ≥ 36hours No official indication for use	Last dose: ≥ 48 hours Last dose: ≥ 48 hours Last dose: ≥ 48 hours Last dose: ≥ 48 hours No official indication for use

longer (at least 36 hours). On the other hand, in high-risk procedures the period of discontinuation should be at least 48 hours.

Taking into consideration that the risk for bleeding complications after some types of surgery may outweigh the risk for thromboembolism, caution is still required (Spyropoulos and Turpie 2005).

NOACs can be resumed postoperatively when adequate haemostasis has been achieved. NOACs should be restarted 6–8 hours after the procedure if immediate and adequate haemostasis has been established (Flaker et al. 2012). In cases of high bleeding risk procedures, full-dose anticoagulation should be postponed by 48–72 hours after the intervention. Prophylactic doses of low-molecular-weight heparin (LMWH) 6–8 hours after the procedure should be considered before restarting NOACs in immobilized patients at high thromboembolic risk if adequate haemostasis has been obtained (Heidbuchel et al. 2013).

6.8 **Cardioversion and ablation in patients treated with NOACs**

It is well established that, in patients with AF of greater than 48 hours' duration (or AF of unknown duration) undergoing cardioversion, therapeutic anticoagulation should have been given for at least 3 weeks prior to and should be continued for 4 weeks after cardioversion.

According to the 2012 update from the ESC, dabigatran represents a valid alternative to warfarin in patients undergoing elective cardioversion (Nagarakanti et al. 2012). Despite the fact that currently there is limited evidence regarding the efficacy and safety profile of rivaroxaban and apixaban in patients undergoing cardioversion, observational data from the RE-LY, ROCKET-AF, and ARISTOTLE trials did not reveal any difference in the rate of strokes or systemic thromboembolic events (Nagarakanti et al. 2011; Flaker et al. 2012; Piccini et al. 2013).

Thus, cardioversion could be considered safe in patients receiving NOACs as long as effective anticoagulation could be reliably confirmed. However, if there is uncertainty concerning the compliance with the anticoagulant treatment it is considered appropriate to perform a transoesophageal echocardiogram in order to exclude the presence of left atrial thrombi. In addition, one study found that ablation performed whilst still receiving dabigatran is associated with increased risk of bleeding or thromboembolic complications compared with uninterrupted warfarin therapy (Lakkireddy et al. 2012).

On the other hand, a recent study using a protocol-based strategy in the periablation setting, revealed that dabigatran has a favourable efficacy and safety profile (Winkle et al. 2012).

One recent study that assessed the use of rivaroxaban in patients with AF undergoing cardioversion or catheter ablation revealed that rivaroxaban seemed to be a safe alternative to warfarin (Piccini et al. 2013).

One new study investigating rivaroxaban use in AF patients undergoing elective cardioversion is currently ongoing. The X-VeRT is the largest randomized study that is expected to assess the efficacy and safety profile of rivaroxaban in comparison to dose-adjusted VKA in the context of elective cardioversion. In addition, VENTURE-AF is a currently ongoing study that is expected to assess the safety profile of rivaroxaban in patients with non-valvular AF undergoing first catheter ablation.

6.9 **'Switch therapy' regimen**

Given the added convenience, the favourable efficacy profile, and safety advantage for fatal bleeding of NOACs, many patients will choose to substitute warfarin for one of the new anticoagulants.

In this setting, warfarin should be interrupted and INR strictly monitored during the following days. It is recommended that dabigatran should be started immediately as soon as the INR falls below 2.0 (Boehringer Ingelheim 2012a, 2012b). When changing from warfarin to rivaroxaban it is recommended that warfarin should be interrupted and rivaroxaban commenced when the INR falls to lower than 3.0 (US labelling) or 2.5 or lower (Canadian label) (Bayer, Inc. 2012; Janssen Pharmaceuticals, Inc. 2012). In cases of conversion from warfarin to apixaban, it is recommended to start apixaban when the INR is lower than 2 (Bristol-Myers Squibb Company 2012a, 2012b).

In the case of conversion from dabigatran to warfarin, the precise time that warfarin should be started is related to renal function. In particular it is suggested that warfarin should be started 3 days before the interruption of dabigatran in case CrCl *is more than 50 mL/min* and 2 days when *CrCl falls between 30 to 50 mL/min* (European Medicines Agency n.d.). Concerning the transition from rivaroxaban to warfarin it is recommended that patients should receive warfarin and a parenteral anticoagulant 24 hours after discontinuation of rivaroxaban (US prescribing information) (Janssen Pharmaceuticals, Inc 2012). Concomitant use of rivaroxaban and warfarin is recommended until INR is at least 2.0 (Bayer, Inc. 2012).

Apixaban should be discontinued and clinicians should start both a parenteral anticoagulant and warfarin at the time the next dose of apixaban would have been taken. The parenteral anticoagulant should be interrupted when INR reaches the target range (Bristol-Myers Squibb Company 2012a). In accordance with Canadian labelling, warfarin should be administrated at usual starting doses and continue apixaban until INR is at least 2, and then apixaban should be interrupted (Bristol-Myers Squibb Company 2012b).

To switch from LMWH to dabigatran, or rivaroxaban it is recommended that dabigatran or rivaroxaban should be administrated 0–2 hours before the time the next dose was scheduled to be given. For patients receiving a continuous infusion UFH, it is recommended that dabigatran or rivaroxaban should be started at the time the infusion is stopped.

If UFH or LMWH is indicated in a patient receiving dabigatran, treatment should be postponed by at least 12 hours after the last dose of dabigatran or until the aPTT is less than 1.5 times the upper limit of normal (European Medicines Agency n.d.). In cases where UFH or LMWH is indicated in a patient treated with rivaroxaban, treatment should be delayed by at least 24 hours after the last dose of rivaroxaban. As far as apixaban is concerned, no recommendations are available at this time in regard to the switch therapy regimen.

6.10 **Post-stenting/acute coronary syndrome anticoagulation**

In the context of acute MI, if there is an indication of percutaneous coronary intervention (PCI) or coronary artery bypass surgery NOACs should be interrupted and patients should be treated according to the current guidelines. If patients are candidates for thrombolysis, it is recommended that patients should undergo coagulation tests (aPTT, triple therapy (TT) and ECT) in order to exclude excess of anticoagulant activity.

In the setting of post stenting/acute coronary syndrome (ACS) the management of AF patients on oral anticoagulation becomes more complex. TT appears the best antithrombotic strategy to prevent both stent thrombosis and thromboembolic complications in AF patients undergoing PCI (Van de Werf et al. 2008). Indeed it is well known that DAPT per se provides suboptimal protection against thromboembolic complications in patients with AF (Rubboli et al. 2005; ACTIVE Writing Group of the ACTIVE Investigators et al. 2006).

On the other hand, TT increases dramatically the risk of bleeding complications. In fact, the overall risk of haemorrhage with TT (warfarin, aspirin, and clopidogrel) was found to be considerably higher (three- to fourfold) than with DAPT (Khurram et al. 2006). Notably in the study by Gao et al. (2010), it was revealed that in patients experiencing bleeding complications on TT, 72% of all the INR measurements were within the target range (1.8–2.5). Additionally the combination of warfarin and aspirin is associated with an almost twofold bleeding risk and the combination of warfarin and clopidogrel with a threefold bleeding risk compared to warfarin monotherapy (Hansen et al. 2010)

Taking also into account not only that the DAPT does not eliminate completely the risk of late stent thrombosis (the rate is about 0.6% per year in patients on DAPT) but also the limitations of VKAs per se to protect patients from stent thrombosis, management of AF patients after the stent implantation is rather complicated and several precautions have to be considered (Daemen et al. 2007).

Risk scores such as the CHA_2DS_2-VASc and the HAS-BLED scores are of crucial importance in order to identify both bleeding and stroke risk in individual patients. A high CHA_2DS_2-VASc score can identify both patients with a high risk for thromboembolic events as well as patients with a high risk for ischaemic heart disease (Van de Werf et al. 2008).

Numerous prospective studies are currently being conducted to evaluate the use of dual and triple therapy in patients with AF undergoing stent implantation. Among them, the MUSICA-2 trial (NCT01141153) and ISAR Triple trial (NCT00776633) are expected to shed light on important aspects of the management strategy of AF patients undergoing PCI. In addition, the phase 3 PIONEER AF-PCI study which will enrol approximately 2100 patients worldwide is designed to assess the safety of two rivaroxaban treatment strategies and a dose-adjusted VKA treatment strategy.

Table 6.7 Antithrombotic strategies following coronary artery stenting in patients with AF			
Low or Intermediate bleeding risk (e.g. HAS-BLED score 0–2)	Elective	Bare-metal	1 month: triple therapy of VKA (INR 2.0–2.5) + aspirin ≤100 mg/day + clopidogrel 75 mg/day Up to 12th month: combination of VKA (INR 2.0–2.5) + clopidogrel 75 mg/day (or aspirin 100 mg/day) Lifelong: VKA (INR 2.0–3.0) alone
	Elective	Drug-eluting	Triple therapy of VKA (INR 2.0–2.5) + aspirin ≤100 mg/day + clopidogrel 75 mg/day Up to 12th month: combination of VKA (INR 2.0–2.5) + clopidogrel 75 mg/day (or aspirin 100 mg/day) Lifelong: VKA (INR 2.0–3.0) alone
	ACS	Bare-metal/ drug-eluting	6 months: triple therapy of VKA (INR 2.0–2.5) + aspirin ≤ 100 mg/day +clopidogrel 75 mg/day Up to 12th month: combination of VKA (INR 2.0–2.5) + clopidogrel 75 mg/day (or aspirin 100 mg/day) Lifelong: VKA (INR 2.0–3.0) alone
High bleeding risk (e.g. HAS-BLED score ≥ 3)	Elective	Bare-metal	2–4 weeks: triple therapy of VKA (INR 2.0–2.5) + aspirin ≤ 100 mg/day + clopidogrel 75 mg/day Lifelong: VKA (INR 2.0–3.0) alone
	ACS	Bare-metal	4 weeks: triple therapy of VKA (INR 2.0–2.5) + aspirin ≤ 100 mg/day + clopidogrel 75 mg/day Up to 12th month: combination of VKA (INR 2.0–2.5) + clopidogrel 75 mg/day (or aspirin 100 mg/day) Lifelong: VKA (INR 2.0–3.0) alone

According to the ESC guidelines the anticoagulation strategy depends on three parameters:

• The bleeding risk (low or intermediate with HAS-BLED score 0–2 or high risk with > 3).

• The clinical setting (elective stenting or ACS).

• Type of stent implanted (bare-metal or drug-eluting).

In essence, the recommended duration of triple therapy varies from 2 weeks to 6 months, and a dual therapy consisting of a vitamin-K-antagonist and clopidogrel is recommended to be used after the triple therapy for up to 12 months after stenting (Table 6.7).

In summary, in patients with AF at moderate to high thromboembolic risk undergoing PCI, TT is generally recommended (Rubboli and Halperin 2008; Rubboli et al. 2012). Individual bleeding risk assessment (as well as strict INR monitoring) is necessary in order for patients to be protected against bleeding complications (Beyth et al. 1998; Guyatt et al. 2012). In addition to that it is essential that use of drug-eluting stents be avoided in patients at high risk of bleeding events so as to shorten the duration of TT. Furthermore the use of proton-pump inhibitors should always be considered in patients on TT, given the high rate of GI haemorrhage (Mattichack et al. 2005; DeEugenio et al. 2007).

Recently, a small randomized trial, the WOEST trial, addressed the issue of DAPT in the setting of post-stenting ACS (Dewilde et al. 2013). WOEST trial showed a large reduction in overall TIMI (Thrombolysis in Myocardial Infarction criteria) bleeding in patients on dual therapy with oral anticoagulants and clopidogrel compared with those receiving TT including aspirin. As far as efficacy is concerned, the WOEST trial concluded that DAPT was not inferior to TT. Although the results of this study are very encouraging and may have an impact on clinical practice, the power of the study in regard to stent thrombosis and stroke was low.

Another important issue raised in the context of post stenting/ACS in AF patients is the role of NOACs. In the RE-LY trial almost 40% of the study population received concomitant aspirin or clopidogrel and almost 5% of patients received DAPT with aspirin and clopidogrel (Eikelboom et al. 2011). A post hoc analysis revealed that in patients receiving concomitant antiplatelet therapy, dabigatran 150 mg twice daily was superior to warfarin in regard to stroke and systemic embolism and equivalent to warfarin in terms of major bleeding. On the other hand, compared with warfarin, dabigatran 110 mg was non-inferior to warfarin relating to stroke and systemic embolism twice a day and was associated with a lower risk of major bleeding. These results were congruent with the main trial results.

In the ARISTOTLE study, subgroup analysis demonstrated that concomitant antiplatelet therapy was not associated with an increased rate of stroke and major bleeding (Raghavan et al. 2009). No subgroup analysis of the ROCKET-AF study addressing this issue is available.

The RE-DEEM study was a phase 2 randomized trial which assessed treatment with an oral anticoagulant added to DAPT, in patients with a recent non-ST or ST-elevation MI. The study showed that the novel oral direct thrombin inhibitor resulted in a low and acceptable bleeding rate (Oldgren et al. 2011) in post-MI patients. Additionally, dabigatran was associated with a decreased cardiovascular event rate. These finding are consistent with the results from APPRAISE and ATLAS phase 2 studies that have evaluated the safety and efficacy of the oral factors Xa inhibitors rivaroxaban and apixaban in combination with DAPT in patients with ACS (Alexander et al. 2011; Mega et al. 2012).

In the phase 3 ATLAS ACS 2–TIMI 51 study, rivaroxaban reduced the risk of the composite endpoint of death from cardiovascular causes, MI, or stroke at the cost of increased major bleeding and intracranial haemorrhage compared to DAPT. In patients with a recent ST segment elevation MI, it was found that rivaroxaban was associated with lower rate of cardiovascular events (Mega et al. 2013).

In the phase 3 APPRAISE-2 study, however, patients were randomized to receive apixaban, or placebo, in addition to mono or dual antiplatelet therapy, but use of apixaban on top of DAPT increased the number of major bleeding events without a significant reduction in recurrent ischaemic events.

On the other hand, novel P2Y12 receptor antagonists, such as prasugrel and ticagrelor, appeared to be superior to clopidogrel regarding major adverse cardiovascular events (Wiviott et al. 2007; Wallentin et al. 2009), at the price of increased major bleeding compared to clopidogrel. Thus, currently TT with OAC, aspirin, and prasugrel/ticagrelor is not recommended because of the higher risk of bleeding.

References

ACTIVE Writing Group of the ACTIVE Investigators, Connolly S, Pogue J, Hart R, Pfeffer M, Hohnloser S, *et al*. Clopidogrel plus aspirin versus oral anticoagulation for atrial fibrillation in the Atrial fibrillation Clopidogrel Trial with Irbesartan for prevention of Vascular Events (ACTIVE W): a randomised controlled trial. *Lancet* 2006; 367: 1903–12.

Alexander JH, Lopes RD, James S, Kilaru R, He Y, Mohan P, *et al*.; APPRAISE-2 Investigators. Apixaban with antiplatelet therapy after acute coronary syndrome. *N Engl J Med* 2011; 365: 699–708.

Apostolakis S, Sullivan RM, Olshansky B, Lip GY. Factors affecting quality of anticoagulation control amongst atrial fibrillation patients on warfarin: The SAMe-TT$_2$R$_2$ score. *Chest* 2013; 144(5): 1555–63.

Artang R, Rome E, Vidaillet H. Dabigatran and myocardial infarction, drug or class effect. Meta-analysis of randomized trials with oral direct thrombin inhibitors. *J Am Coll Cardiol* 2012; 59: E571.

Avgil Tsadok M, Jackevicius CA, Rahme E, Humphries KH, Behlouli H, Pilote L. Sex differences in stroke risk among older patients with recently diagnosed atrial fibrillation. *JAMA* 2012; 307: 1952–8.

Barrett YC, Wang Z, Frost C, Shenker A. Clinical laboratory measurement of direct factor Xa inhibitors: anti-Xa assay is preferable to prothrombin time assay. *Thromb Haemost* 2010; 104(6): 1263–71.

Bayer, Inc. *Product monograph for Xarelto.* Toronto, ON: Bayer Inc. July 2012. Available at: <http://www.bayer.ca/files/XARELTO-PM-ENG-28AUG2013-164839.pdf>.

Benjamin EJ, Levy D, Vaziri SM, D'Agostino RB, Belanger AJ, Wolf PA. Independent risk factors for atrial fibrillation in a population-based cohort. the Framingham Heart Study. *JAMA* 1994; 271: 840–4.

Beyth RJ, Quinn LM, Landefeld CS. Prospective evaluation of an index for predicting the risk of major bleeding in outpatients treated with warfarin. *Am J Med* 1998; 105: 91–9.

Birman-Deych E, Radford MJ, Nilasena DS, Gage BF. Use and effectiveness of warfarin in Medicare beneficiaries with atrial fibrillation. *Stroke* 2006; 37: 1070–4.

Blech S, Ebner T, Ludwig-Schwellinger E, Stangier J, Roth W. The metabolism and disposition of the oral direct thrombin inhibitor, dabigatran, in humans. *Drug Metab Dispos* 2008; 36: 386–99.

Boehringer Ingelheim. *Product information for Pradaxa.* Ridgefield, CT: Boehringer Ingelheim Pharmaceuticals, Inc. December 2012a.

Boehringer Ingelheim. *Product monograph for Pradaxa.* Boehringer Ingelheim Canada Ltd. Burlington, ON: Boehringer Ingelheim Canada Ltd. December 2012b.

Bristol-Myers Squibb Company. *Product information for Eliquis.* Princeton, NJ: Bristol-Myers Squibb Company. December 2012a.

Bristol-Myers Squibb Company. *Product monograph for Eliquis.* Montreal, QC: Bristol-Myers Squibb Canada. November 2012b.

Bungard TJ, Ghali WA, Teo KK, McAlister FA, Tsuyuki RT. Why do patients with atrial fibrillation not receive warfarin? *Arch Intern Med* 2000; 160: 41–6.

Camm AJ, Kirchhof P, Lip GY, Schotten U, Savelieva I, Ernst S, *et al.* European Heart Rhythm Association, European Association for Cardio-Thoracic Surgery. Guidelines for the management of atrial fibrillation. The Task Force for the management of atrial fibrillation of the European society of Cardiology (ESC). *Eur Heart J* 2010; 31: 2369–429

Camm AJ, Lip GY, De Caterina R, Savelieva I, Atar D, Hohnloser SH, *et al.* 2012 focused update of the ESC Guidelines for the management of atrial fibrillation: an update of the 2010 ESC Guidelines for the management of atrial fibrillation. Developed with the special contribution of the European Heart Rhythm Association. *Eur Heart J* 2012; 33(21): 2719–47.

Connolly SJ, Eikelboom J, Joyner C, Diener HC, Hart R, Golitsyn S, *et al.*; AVERROES Steering Committee and Investigators. Apixaban in patients with atrial fibrillation. *N Engl J Med* 2011; 364: 806–17.

Connolly SJ, Ezekowitz MD, Yusuf S, Eikelboom J, Oldgren J, Parekh A, *et al.*; RE-LY Steering Committee and Investigators. Dabigatran vs. warfarin in patients with atrial fibrillation. *N Engl J Med* 2009a; 361: 1139–51.

Connolly SJ, Ezekowitz MD, Yusuf S, Reilly PA, Wallentin L. Newly identified events in the RE-LY trial. *N Engl J Med* 2010; 363: 1875–6.

Connolly SJ, Pogue J, Eikelboom J, Flaker G, Commerford P, Franzosi MG, Healey JS, Yusuf S; ACTIVE W Investigators. Benefit of oral anticoagulant over antiplatelet therapy in atrial fibrillation depends on the quality of international normalized ratio control achieved by centers and countries as measured by time in therapeutic range. *Circulation* 2008; 118(20): 2029–37.

Connolly SJ, Pogue J, Hart RG, Hohnloser SH, Pfeffer M, Chrolavicius S, Yusuf S. Effect of clopidogrel added to aspirin in patients with atrial fibrillation. *N Engl J Med* 2009b; 360: 2066–78.

Connolly SJ, Wallentin L, Ezekowitz MD, Eikelboom JW, Oldgren J, Reilly PA, *et al.* The Long Term Multi-Center Observational Study of Dabigatran Treatment in Patients with Atrial Fibrillation: (RELY-ABLE) Study. *Circulation* 2013; 128(3): 237–43.

Daemen J, Wenaweser P, Tsuchida K, Abrecht L, Vaina S, Morger C, *et al.* Early and late coronary stent thrombosis of sirolimus-eluting and paclitaxel-eluting stents in routine clinical practice: data from a large two-institutional cohort study. *Lancet* 2007; 369: 667–78.

DeEugenio D, Kolman L, DeCaro M, Andrel J, Chervoneva I, Duong P, *et al.* Risk of major bleeding with concomitant dual antiplatelet therapy after percutaneous coronary intervention in patients receiving long-term warfarin therapy. *Pharmacotherapy* 2007, 27: 691–6.

Deitelzweig S, Amin A, Jing Y, Makenbaeva D, Wiederkehr D, Lin J, Graham J. Medical cost reductions associated with the usage of novel oral anticoagulants vs warfarin among atrial fibrillation patients, based on the RE-LY, ROCKET-AF, and ARISTOTLE trials. *J Med Econ* 2012; 15: 776–85.

Devereux RB, Roman MJ, Paranicas M, O'Grady MJ, Lee ET, Welty TK, *et al.* Impact of diabetes on cardiac structure and function: the strong heart study. *Circulation* 2000; 101: 2271–6.

Dewilde WJ, Oirbans T, Verheugt FW, Kelder JC, De Smet BJ, Herrman JP, *et al.*; WOEST study investigators. Use of clopidogrel with or without aspirin in patients taking oral anticoagulant therapy and undergoing percutaneous coronary intervention: an open-label, randomised, controlled trial. *Lancet* 2013; 381: 1107–15.

Eby C. Novel anticoagulants and laboratory testing. *Int J Lab Hematol* 2013; 35: 262–8.

Eikelboom JW, Wallentin L, Connolly SJ, Ezekowitz M, Healey JS, Oldgren J, *et al.* Risk of bleeding with 2 doses of dabigatran compared with warfarin in older and younger patients with atrial fibrillation: an analysis of the randomized evaluation of long-term anticoagulant therapy (RE-LY) trial. *Circulation* 2011; 123: 2363–72.

European Medicines Agency. *Pradaxa. Summary of product characteristics.* Available at: <http://www.ema.europa.eu/docs/en_GB/document_library/EPAR_-_Product_Information/human/000829/WC500041059.pdf>.

Flaker G, Lopes R, Al-Khatib S, Hermosillo A, Thomas L, Zhu J, Ruzyllo W, Mohan P, Granger C. Apixaban and warfarin are associated with a low risk of stroke following cardioversion for AF: results from the ARISTOTLE Trial. *Eur Heart J* 2012; 33: 686.

Fleming TR, Emerson SS. Evaluating rivaroxaban for atrial fibrillation: regulatory considerations. *N Engl J Med* 2011; 365: 1557–9.

Food and Drug Administration. *Xarelto (rivaroxaban). Prescribing information.* 2013. Available at: <http://www.accessdata.fda.gov/drugsatfda_docs/label/2013/022406s004lbl.pdf>.

Freeman JV, Zhu RP, Owens DK, Garber AM, Hutton DW, Go AS, *et al.* Cost-effectiveness of dabigatran compared with warfarin for stroke prevention in atrial fibrillation. *Ann Intern Med* 2011; 154: 1–11.

Friberg L, Rosenqvist M, Lip GY. Net clinical benefit of warfarin in patients with atrial fibrillation: a report from the Swedish atrial fibrillation cohort study. *Circulation* 2012; 125: 2298–307.

Gage BF, Waterman AD, Shannon W, Boechler M, Rich MW, Radford MJ. Validation of clinical classification schemes for predicting stroke: results from the National Registry of Atrial Fibrillation. *JAMA* 2001; 285: 2864–70.

Gao F, Zhou YJ, Wang ZJ, Shen H, Liu XL, Nie B, Yan ZX, Yang SW, Jia de A, Yu M. Comparison of different antithrombotic regimens for patients with atrial fibrillation undergoing drug-eluting stent implantation. *Circ J* 2010; 74: 701–8.

Go AS, Hylek EM, Borowsky LH, Phillips KA, Selby JV, Singer DE. Warfarin use among ambulatory patients with non-valvular atrial fibrillation: the AnTicoagulation and Risk Factors in Atrial Fibrillation (ATRIA) Study. *Ann Intern Med* 1999; 131: 927–34.

Go AS, Hylek EM, Phillips KA, Chang Y, Henault LE, Selby JV, Singer DE. Prevalence of diagnosed atrial fibrillation in adults: national implications for rhythm management and stroke prevention: the AnTicoagulation and Risk Factors in Atrial Fibrillation (ATRIA) Study. *JAMA* 2001; 285: 2370–5.

Goette A, Bukowska A, Dobrev D, Pfeiffenberger J, Morawietz H, Strugala D, *et al.* Acute atrial tachyarrhythmia induces angiotensin II type 1 receptor-mediated oxidative stress and microvascular flow abnormalities in the ventricles. *Eur Heart J* 2009; 30: 1411–20.

Gorin L, Fauchier L, Nonin E, de Labriolle A, Haguenoer K, Cosnay P, *et al.* Antithrombotic treatment and the risk of death and stroke in patients with atrial fibrillation and a CHADS2 score=1. *Thromb Haemost* 2010; 103: 833–40.

Granger CB, Alexander JH, McMurray JJ, Lopes RD, Hylek EM, Hanna M *et al.* ARISTOTLE Committees and Investigators. Apixaban versus warfarin in patients with atrial fibrillation. *N Engl J Med.* 2011; 365(11): 981–92.

Guyatt GH, Akl EA, Crowther M, Gutterman DD, Schünemann HJ; American College of Chest Physicians Antithrombotic Therapy and Prevention of Thrombosis Panel. Executive summary: Antithrombotic Therapy and Prevention of Thrombosis, 9th ed: American College of Chest Physicians Evidence-Based Clinical Practice Guidelines. *Chest* 2012; 141: 7S–47S.

Hansen ML, Sørensen R, Clausen MT, Fog-Petersen ML, Raunsø J, Gadsbøll N, *et al.* Risk of bleeding with single, dual, or triple therapy with warfarin, aspirin, and clopidogrel in patients with atrial fibrillation. *Arch Intern Med* 2010; 170: 1433–41.

Hart RG, Benavente O, McBride R, Pearce LA. Antithrombotic therapy to prevent stroke in patients with atrial fibrillation: a meta-analysis. *Ann Intern Med* 1999; 131: 492–501.

Hart RG, Pearce LA, Aguilar MI. Meta-analysis: antithrombotic therapy to prevent stroke in patients who have nonvalvular atrial fibrillation. *Ann Intern Med* 2007; 146: 857–67.

Hauel NH, Nar H, Priepke H, Ries U, Stassen JM, Wienen W. Structure-based design of novel potent nonpeptide thrombin inhibitors. *J Med Chem* 2002; 45: 1757–66.

Heeringa J, van der Kuip DA, Hofman A, Kors JA, van Herpen G, Stricker BH, *et al*. Prevalence, incidence and lifetime risk of atrial fibrillation: the Rotterdam study. *Eur Heart J* 2006; 27: 949–53.

Heidbuchel H, Verhamme P, Alings M, Antz M, Hacke W, Oldgren J, *et al*. EHRA Practical Guide on the use of new oral anticoagulants in patients with non-valvular atrial fibrillation: executive summary. *Eur Heart J* 2013; 34: 2094–106.

Hnatkova K, Waktare JE, Murgatroyd FD, Guo X, Camm AJ, Malik M. Age and gender influences on rate and duration of paroxysmal atrial fibrillation. *Pacing Clin Electrophysiol* 1998; 21: 2455–8.

Hughes M, Lip GY. Stroke and thromboembolism in atrial fibrillation: a systematic review of stroke risk factors, risk stratification schema and cost effectiveness data. *Thromb Haemost* 2008; 99: 295–304.

Huisman MV, Lip GY, Diener HC, Brueckmann M, van Ryn J, Clemens A. Dabigatran etexilate for stroke prevention in patients with atrial fibrillation: resolving uncertainties in routine practice. *Thromb Haemost* 2012; 107: 838–47.

Humphries KH, Kerr CR, Connolly SJ, Klein G, Boone JA, Green M, *et al*. New-onset atrial fibrillation: sex differences in presentation, treatment, and outcome. *Circulation* 2001; 103: 2365–70.

Hutchaleelaha A, Lu G, Deguzman FR, Karbarz MJ, Inagaki M, Yau S, *et al.* Recombinant factor Xa inhibitor antidote (PRT064445) mediates reversal of anticoagulation through reduction of free drug concentration: a common mechanism for direct factor Xa inhibitors. ESC Congress 2012. *Eur Heart J* 2012; 33(Abstract Supplement), 496.

Hylek EM, D'Antonio J, Evans-Molina C, Shea C, Henault LE, Regan S. Translating the results of randomized trials into clinical practice: the challenge of warfarin candidacy among hospitalized elderly patients with atrial fibrillation. *Stroke* 2006; 37: 1075–80.

Hylek EM, Evans-Molina C, Shea C, Henault LE, Regan S. Major hemorrhage and tolerability of warfarin in the first year of therapy among elderly patients with atrial fibrillation. *Circulation* 2007; 115: 2689–96.

Hylek EM, Go AS, Chang Y, Jensvold NG, Henault LE, Selby JV, Singer DE. Effect of intensity of oral anticoagulation on stroke severity and mortality in atrial fibrillation. *N Engl J Med* 2003; 349: 1019–26.

Janssen Pharmaceuticals, Inc. *Product information for Xarelto*. Titusville, NJ: Janssen Pharmaceuticals, Inc. November 2012.

Kanagala R, Murali NS, Friedman PA, Ammash NM, Gersh BJ, Ballman KV, *et al*. Obstructive sleep apnea and the recurrence of atrial fibrillation. *Circulation* 2003; 107: 2589–94.

Kannel WB, Abbott RD, Savage DD, McNamara PM. Epidemiologic features of chronic atrial fibrillation: the Framingham study. *N Engl J Med* 1982; 306: 1018–22.

Kannel WB, Benjamin EJ. Final draft status of the epidemiology of atrial fibrillation. *Med Clin North Am* 2008; 92: 17–40.

Kannel WB, Wolf PA, Benjamin EJ, Levy D. Prevalence, incidence, prognosis, and predisposing conditions for atrial fibrillation: population-based estimates. *Am J Cardiol* 1998; 82: 2N–9N.

Kansal AR, Sharma M, Bradley-Kennedy C, Clemens A, Monz BU, Peng S, *et al*. Dabigatran versus rivaroxaban for the prevention of stroke and systemic embolism in atrial fibrillation in Canada. Comparative efficacy and cost-effectiveness. *Thromb Haemost* 2012; 108: 672–82.

Kerr C, Boone J, Connolly S, Greene M, Klein G, Sheldon R, Talajic M. Follow-up of atrial fibrillation: The initial experience of the Canadian Registry of Atrial Fibrillation. *Eur Heart J* 1996; 17(Suppl C): 48–51.

Khan AM, Lubitz SA, Sullivan LM, Sun JX, Levy D, Vasan RS, *et al*. Low serum magnesium and the development of atrial fibrillation in the community: the Framingham Heart Study. *Circulation* 2013; 127: 33–8.

Khurram Z, Chou E, Minutello R, Bergman G, Parikh M, Naidu S, *et al*. Combination therapy with aspirin, clopidogrel and warfarin following coronary stenting is associated with a significant risk of bleeding. *J Invasive Cardiol* 2006; 18: 162–4.

Kirchhof P, Auricchio A, Bax J, Crijns H, Camm J, Diener HC, *et al*. Outcome parameters for trials in atrial fibrillation: executive summary. *Eur Heart J* 2007; 28: 2803–17.

Krahn AD, Manfreda J, Tate RB, Mathewson FA, Cuddy TE. The natural history of atrial fibrillation: incidence, risk factors, and prognosis in the Manitoba Follow-Up Study. *Am J Med* 1995; 98: 476–84.

Lakkireddy D, Reddy YM, Di Biase L, Vanga SR, Santangeli P, Swarup V, *et al.* Feasibility and safety of dabigatran versus warfarin for periprocedural anticoagulation in patients undergoing radiofrequency ablation for atrial fibrillation: results from a multicenter prospective registry. *J Am Coll Cardiol* 2012; 59: 1168–74.

Larsen TB, Rasmussen LH, Skjøth F, Due KM, Callréus T, Rosenzweig M, *et al.* Efficacy and safety of dabigatran etexilate and warfarin in 'real-world' patients with atrial fibrillation: a prospective nationwide cohort study. *J Am Coll Cardiol* 2013; 61: 2264–73.

Laupacis A, Albers G, Dunn M, Feinberg W. Antithrombotic therapy in atrial fibrillation. *Chest* 1992; 102(Suppl 4): 426S–433S.

Lee S, Anglade MW, Pham D, Pisacane R, Kluger J, Coleman CI. Cost-effectiveness of rivaroxaban compared to warfarin for stroke prevention in atrial fibrillation. *Am J Cardiol* 2012; 110: 845–51.

Lin HJ, Wolf PA, Kelly-Hayes M, Beiser AS, Kase CS, Benjamin EJ, D'Agostino RB. Stroke severity in atrial fibrillation. The Framingham Study. *Stroke* 1996; 27: 1760–4.

Lip GY, Golding DJ, Nazir M, Beevers DG, Child DL, Fletcher RI. A survey of atrial fibrillation in general practice: the West Birmingham Atrial Fibrillation Project. *Br J Gen Pract* 1997; 47(418): 285–9.

Lip GY, Halperin JL. Improving stroke risk stratification in atrial fibrillation. *Am J Med* 2010; 123: 484–8.

Lip GY, Lane DA. Does warfarin for stroke thromboprophylaxis protect against MI in atrial fibrillation patients? *Am J Med* 2010; 123: 785–9.

Lip GY, Larsen TB, Skjøth F, Rasmussen LH. Indirect comparisons of new oral anticoagulant drugs for efficacy and safety when used for stroke prevention in atrial fibrillation. *J Am Coll Cardiol* 2012; 60(8): 738–46.

Lip GY, Nieuwlaat R, Pisters R, Lane DA, Crijns HJ. Refining clinical risk stratification for predicting stroke and thromboembolism in atrial fibrillation using a novel risk factor-based approach: the euro heart survey on atrial fibrillation. *Chest* 2010; 137: 263–72.

Lloyd-Jones DM, Wang TJ, Leip EP, Larson MG, Levy D, Vasan RS, *et al.* Lifetime risk for development of atrial fibrillation: the Framingham Heart Study. *Circulation* 2004; 110: 1042–6.

Lu G, DeGuzman FR, Hollenbach SJ, Karbarz MJ, Abe K, Lee G, *et al.* A specific antidote for reversal of anticoagulation by direct and indirect inhibitors of coagulation factor Xa. *Nat Med* 2013; 19: 446–51

Mantha S, Ansell J. An indirect comparison of dabigatran, rivaroxaban and apixaban for atrial fibrillation. *Thromb Haemost* 2012; 108: 476–84.

Marini C, De Santis F, Sacco S, Russo T, Olivieri L, Totaro R, Carolei A. Contribution of atrial fibrillation to incidence and outcome of ischaemic stroke: results from a population-based study. *Stroke* 2005; 36: 1115–19.

Marinigh R, Lane DA, Lip GY Severe renal impairment and stroke prevention in atrial fibrillation: implications for thromboprophylaxis and bleeding risk. *J Am Coll Cardiol* 2011; 57: 1339–48.

Maron BJ, Towbin JA, Thiene G, Antzelevitch C, Corrado D, Arnett D, *et al.* Contemporary definitions and classification of the cardiomyopathies: an American Heart Association Scientific Statement from the Council on Clinical Cardiology, Heart Failure and Transplantation Committee; Quality of Care and Outcomes Research and Functional Genomics and Translational Biology Interdisciplinary Working Groups; and Council on Epidemiology and Prevention. *Circulation* 2006; 113: 1807–16

Matchar DB, McCroy DC, Barnett HJM, Feussner JR. Guidelines for medical treatment for stroke prevention. *Ann Intern Med* 1994; 121: 54–5.

Mattichack SJ, Reed PS, Gallagher MJ, Boura JA, O'Neill WW, Kahn JK. Evaluation of safety of warfarin in combination with antiplatelet therapy for patients treated with coronary stents for acute myocardial infarction. *J Interven Cardiol* 2005, 18: 163–6.

Mega JL, Braunwald E, Murphy SA, Plotnikov AN, Burton P, Kiss RG, *et al.* Rivaroxaban in patients stabilized after a ST-segment elevation myocardial infarction: results from the ATLAS ACS-2-TIMI-51 trial (Anti-Xa Therapy to Lower Cardiovascular Events in Addition to Standard Therapy in Subjects with Acute Coronary Syndrome-Thrombolysis In Myocardial Infarction-51). *J Am Coll Cardiol* 2013; 6118: 1853–9.

Mega JL, Braunwald E, Wiviott SD, Bassand JP, Bhatt DL, Bode C, *et al.*; ATLAS ACS 2–TIMI 51 Investigators. Rivaroxaban in patients with a recent acute coronary syndrome. *N Engl J Med* 2012; 366: 9–19.

Miyasaka Y, Barnes ME, Gersh BJ, Cha SS, Bailey KR, Abhayaratna WP, et al. Secular trends in incidence of atrial fibrillation in Olmsted County, Minnesota, 1980 to 2000, and implications on the projections for future prevalence. *Circulation* 2006; 114: 119–25.

Morley J, Marinchak R, Rials SJ, Kowey P. Atrial fibrillation, anticoagulation, and stroke. *Am J Cardiol* 1996; 77(3): 38A–44A.

Nabauer M, Gerth A, Limbourg T, Schneider S, Oeff M, Kirchhof P, et al. The Registry of the German Competence NETwork on Atrial Fibrillation: patient characteristics and initial management. *Europace* 2009; 11: 423–34.

Naccarelli GV, Varker H, Lin J, Schulman KL. Increasing prevalence of atrial fibrillation and flutter in the United States. *Am J Cardiol* 2009; 104: 1534–9.

Nagarakanti R, Ezekowitz MD, Oldgren J, Yang S, Chernick M, Aikens TH, et al. Dabigatran versus warfarin in patients with atrial fibrillation: an analysis of patients undergoing cardioversion. *Circulation* 2011; 123: 131–6.

Nieuwlaat R, Capucci A, Camm AJ, Olsson SB, Andresen D, Davies DW, et al; European Heart Survey Investigators. Atrial fibrillation management: a prospective survey in ESC member countries: the Euro Heart Survey on Atrial Fibrillation. *Eur Heart J* 2005; 26: 2422–34.

Nieuwlatt R, Capucci A, Lip GYH, Olsson SB, Prins MH, Nieman FH, et al.; on behalf of the Euro Heart Survey Investigators. Antithrombotic treatment in real-life atrial fibrillation patients: a report from the Euro Heart Survey on Atrial Fibrillation. *Eur Heart J* 2006; 27: 3018–26.

Oldgren J, Budaj A, Granger CB, Khder Y, Roberts J, Siegbahn A, et al.; RE-DEEM Investigators. Dabigatran vs. placebo in patients with acute coronary syndromes on dual antiplatelet therapy: a randomized, double-blind, phase II trial. *Eur Heart J* 2011; 32: 2781–9.

Olesen JB, Lip GY, Lindhardsen J, Lane DA, Ahlehoff O, Hansen ML, et al. Risks of thromboembolism and bleeding with thromboprophylaxis in patients with atrial fibrillation: a net clinical benefit analysis using a 'real world' nationwide cohort study. *Thromb Haemost* 2011; 106: 739–49.

Park H, Hildreth A, Thomson R, O'Connell J. Non-valvular atrial fibrillation and cognitive decline: a longitudinal cohort study. *Age Ageing* 2007; 36: 157–63.

Patel MR, Mahaffey KW, Garg J, Pan G, Singer DE, Hacke W, et al.; ROCKET AF Investigators. Rivaroxaban vs. warfarin in nonvalvular atrial fibrillation. *N Engl J Med* 2011; 365: 883–91.

Piccini JP, Stevens SR, Lokhnygina Y, Patel MR, Halperin JL, Singer DE, et al; ROCKET AF Steering Committee & Investigators. Outcomes after cardioversion and atrial fibrillation ablation in patients treated with rivaroxaban and warfarin in the ROCKET AF trial. *J Am Coll Cardiol* 2013; 61(19): 1998–2006.

Pink J, Lane S, Pirmohamed M, Hughes DA. Dabigatran etexilate versus warfarin in management of non-valvular atrial fibrillation in UK context: quantitative benefit-harm and economic analyses. *BMJ* 2011 31; 343: d6333.

Pisters R, Lane DA, Nieuwlaat R, de Vos CB, Crijns HJ, Lip GY. A novel user-friendly score (HAS-BLED) to assess 1-year risk of major bleeding in patients with atrial fibrillation: the Euro Heart Survey. *Chest* 2010; 138: 1093–100.

Raghavan N, Frost CE, Yu Z, He K, Zhang H, Humphreys WG, et al. Apixaban metabolism and pharmacokinetics after oral administration to humans. *Drug Metab Dispos* 2009; 37: 74–81.

Rasmussen LH, Larsen TB, Graungaard T, Skjøth F, Lip GY. Primary and secondary prevention with new oral anticoagulant drugs for stroke prevention in atrial fibrillation: indirect comparison analysis. *BMJ* 2012; 345: e7097.

Rastas S, Verkkoniemi A, Polvikoski T, Juva K, Niinistö L, Mattila K, et al. Atrial fibrillation, stroke, and cognition. A longitudinal population-based study of people aged 85 and older. *Stroke* 2007; 38: 1454–60.

Rubboli A, Halperin JL. Pro: 'Antithrombotic therapy with warfarin, aspirin and clopidogrel is the recommended regime in anticoagulated patients who present with an acute coronary syndrome and/or undergo percutaneous coronary interventions'. *Thromb Haemost* 2008; 100: 752–3.

Rubboli A, Magnavacchi P, Guastaroba P, Saia F, Vignali L, Giacometti P, et al. Antithrombotic management and 1-year outcome of patients on oral anticoagulation undergoing coronary stent implantation (from the Registro Regionale Angioplastiche Emilia-Romagna Registry). *Am J Cardiol* 2012; 109: 1411–17.

Rubboli A, Milandri M, Castelvetri C, Cosmi B: Meta-analysis of trials comparing oral anticoagulation and aspirin versus dual antiplatelet therapy after coronary stenting. Clues for the management of

125

patients with an indication for long-term anticoagulation undergoing coronary stenting. *Cardiology* 2005, 104: 101–6.

Samama MM, Guinet C. Laboratory assessment of new anticoagulants. *Clin Chem Lab Med* 2011; 49: 761–72.

Sato H, Ishikawa K, Kitabatake A, Ogawa S, Maruyama Y, Yokota Y, *et al.* Low-dose aspirin for prevention of stroke in low-risk patients with atrial fibrillation: Japan Atrial Fibrillation Stroke Trial. *Stroke* 2006; 37: 447–51.

Schulz R, Eisele HJ, Seeger W. Nocturnal atrial fibrillation in a patient with obstructive sleep apnoea. *Thorax* 2005; 60: 174.

Shah SV, Gage BF. Cost-effectiveness of dabigatran for stroke prophylaxis in atrial fibrillation. *Circulation* 2011; 123: 2562–70.

Sorensen SV, Kansal AR, Connolly S, Peng S, Linnehan J, Bradley-Kennedy C, Plumb JM. Cost-effectiveness of dabigatran etexilate for the prevention of stroke and systemic embolism in atrial fibrillation: a Canadian payer perspective. *Thromb Haemost* 2011; 105: 908–19.

Spyropoulos AC, Turpie AG. Perioperative bridging interruption with heparin for the patient receiving long-term anticoagulation. *Curr Opin Pulm Med* 2005; 11(5): 373–9.

Stangier J, Eriksson BI, Dahl OE, Ahnfelt L, Nehmiz G, Stähle H, *et al.* Pharmacokinetic profile of the oral direct thrombin inhibitor dabigatran etexilate in healthy volunteers and patients undergoing total hip replacement. *J Clin Pharmacol* 2005; 45: 555–63.

Stangier J, Feuring M. Using the HEMOCLOT direct thrombin inhibitor assay to determine plasma concentrations of dabigatran. *Blood Coagul Fibrinolysis* 2012; 23: 138–43.

Stangier J, Rathgen K, Stähle H, Gansser D, Roth W. The pharmacokinetics, pharmacodynamics and tolerability of dabigatran etexilate, a new oral direct thrombin inhibitor, in healthy male subjects. *Br J Clin Pharmacol* 2007; 64: 292–303.

Stangier J, Rathgen K, Stähle H, Mazur D. Influence of renal impairment on the pharmacokinetics and pharmacodynamics of oral dabigatran etexilate: an open-label, parallel-group, single-centre study. *Clin Pharmacokinet* 2010; 49: 259–68.

Stewart S, Hart CL, Hole DJ, McMurray JJ. A population-based study of the longterm risks associated with atrial fibrillation: 20-year follow-up of the Renfrew/ Paisley study. *Am J Med* 2002; 113: 359–64.

Stritzke J, Markus MR, Duderstadt S, Lieb W, Luchner A, Döring A, *et al.*; MONICA/KORA Investigators. The aging process of the heart: obesity is the main risk factor for left atrial enlargement during aging the MONICA/KORA (monitoring of trends and determinations in cardiovascular disease/cooperative research in the region of Augsburg) study. *J Am Coll Cardiol* 2009; 54: 1982–9.

Stroke Risk in Atrial Fibrillation Working Group. Independent predictors of stroke in patients with atrial fibrillation: a systematic review. *Neurology* 2007; 69: 546–54.

Tikoff G, Schmidt AM, Hecht HH. Atrial fibrillation in atrial septal defect. *Arch Intern Med* 1968; 121: 402–5.

Tripodi A. Measuring the anticoagulant effect of direct factor Xa inhibitors.Is the anti-Xa assay preferable to the prothrombin time test? *Thromb Haemost* 2011; 105: 735–6.

Van de Werf F, Bax J, Betriu A, Blomstrom-Lundqvist C, Crea F, Falk V, *et al.*; ESC Committee for Practice Guidelines (CPG). Management of acute myocardial infarction in patients presenting with persistent ST-segment elevation: the Task Force on the Management of ST-Segment Elevation Acute Myocardial Infarction of the European Society of Cardiology. *Eur Heart J* 2008; 29: 2909–45.

Van Ryn J, Stangier J, Haertter S, Liesenfeld KH, Wienen W, Feuring M, Clemens A. Dabigatran etexilate—a novel, reversible, oral direct thrombin inhibitor: interpretation of coagulation assays and reversal of anticoagulant activity. *Thromb Haemost* 2010; 103: 1116–27.

Van Ryn J, Hauel N, Waldmann L, Wienen W. Dabigatran inhibits both clot-bound and fluid phase thrombin *in vitro*: effects compared to heparin and hirudin. *Blood* 2007; 110: 3998.

Waldo AL, Becker RC, Tapson VF, Colgan KJ; for the NABOR Steering Committee. Hospitalized patients with atrial fibrillation and a high risk of stroke are not being provided with adequate anticoagulation. *J Am Coll Cardiol* 2005; 46: 1729–36.

Wallentin L, Becker RC, Budaj A, Cannon CP, Emanuelsson H, Held C, *et al.*, for the PLATO Investigators. Ticagrelor versus clopidogrel in patients with acute coronary syndromes. *N Engl J Med* 2009; 361: 1045–57.

Warkentin TE, Margetts P, Connolly SJ, Lamy A, Ricci C, Eikelboom JW. Recombinant factor VIIa (rFVIIa) and hemodialysis to manage massive dabigatran-associated postcardiac surgery bleeding. *Blood* 2012; 119: 2172–4.

Wattigney WA, Mensah GA, Croft JB. Increasing trends in hospitalization for atrial fibrillation in the United States, 1985 through 1999: implications for primary prevention. *Circulation* 2003; 108: 711–16.

Wienen W, Stassen JM, Priepke H, Ries UJ, Hauel N. In-vitro profile andex-vivo anticoagulant activity of the direct thrombin inhibitor dabigatran and its orally active prodrug, dabigatran etexilate. *Thromb Haemost* 2007; 98: 155–62.

Winkle RA, Mead RH, Engel G, Kong MH, Patrawala RA. The use of dabigatran immediately after atrial fibrillation ablation. *J Cardiovasc Electrophysiol* 2012; 23(3): 264–8.

Wiviott S, Braunwald E, McCabe C, Montalescot G, Ruzyllo W, Gottlieb S, *et al.* Prasugrel versus clopidogrel in patients with acute coronary syndromes. *N Engl J Med* 2007; 357: 2001–15.

Chapter 7

When to refer patients for non-pharmacological therapies

L. Brent Mitchell

Key points

- Non-pharmacological alternatives exist to accomplish each of the therapeutic goals of treatment of the patient with atrial fibrillation (AF).

- AF ventricular response rate control may be achieved by the ablate-and-pace approach where the AV junction is ablated to produce AV block allowing the ventricular rate to be controlled by an implanted pacemaker.

- AF rhythm control may be achieved by surgical or catheter ablation of AF triggers and/or AF maintenance substrates.

- Implantable device therapy for prevention or rapid termination of AF has only achieved significant success in patients with an independent indication for a pacemaker.

- Surgical or transcatheter occlusion of the left atrial appendage is emerging as an alternative to chronic anticoagulation therapy for prevention of AF-related thromboembolic events and stroke.

129

7.1 Introduction to non-pharmacological treatments for atrial fibrillation

In addition to therapies directed at the cause of atrial fibrillation (AF), including those designed to optimize cardiac structure and function, other therapies for the patient with AF include intermittent or continuous drug treatments for ventricular response rate control, for atrial tachyarrhythmia rhythm control, and for the prevention of thromboembolic events including stroke. Each of these pharmacological approaches has a non-pharmacological surgical or catheter-based alternative.

7.2 The ablate-and-pace approach

The ventricular response rate to AF can be controlled by catheter ablation of the atrioventricular (AV) junction to create purposeful third-degree AV block. Usually, the compact portion of the AV node is targeted from the septal right atrium at the apex of the triangle of Koch approximately 0.8 cm posterior and 0.8 cm inferior to the His bundle recording site. Less commonly, an atrial transseptal puncture is required to allow the His bundle to be targeted from the septal left ventricle. In most patients, the subsequent escape rhythm is junctional at approximately 40 beats per minute (bpm). Accordingly, ventricular pacing is also required. For patients with persistent or permanent AF, a VVIR pacemaker is usually placed prior to the AV junction ablation procedure. For patients with paroxysmal AF, a DDD pacing system may be used in the (unsubstantiated) hope that such pacing will delay the progression of paroxysmal AF to permanent AF.

The major advantage of the ablate-and-pace approach is that it is almost always successful at controlling the ventricular response rate to AF and controlling symptoms related to rapid or irregular ventricular responses thereby permitting the discontinuation of medications used for this purpose.

The major disadvantage of the ablate-and-pace approach is that pacing is then required. Some patients lack a reliable escape rhythm after the ablation and are completely pacemaker dependent. This outcome is more likely in the elderly, with more distal AV conduction system ablation (i.e. His bundle ablation), and when AV nodal conduction suppressant medications are used and is apparent only after the ablation has been performed. Patients adapted to a rapid ventricular rate in AF may respond to sudden slowing of their ventricular response with torsade de pointes ventricular tachycardia and a small risk of sudden death. This possibility is addressed by pacing faster than normal (approximately 80–90 bpm) with slowing of the pacing rate over the few months after the ablation leaving a persisting risk of sudden death that is not different than that of other AF patients. Other disadvantages of the ablate-and-pace approach include its irreversibility, continuation of AF and the need for anticoagulation in many patients, absent AV synchrony, and the potential for right ventricular pacing to exacerbate heart failure by causing ventricular dyssynchrony. Nevertheless, the latter consequence can be overcome with biventricular pacing. Indeed, placement of a biventricular pacing system should be considered in patients with left ventricular (LV) systolic dysfunction thought not to be due to a tachycardiomyopathy prior to the ablation.

Partial ablation of the AV conduction system to prolong AV nodal refractoriness without producing heart block and the need for permanent pacing has also been proposed. The inferior input to the AV node, the slow AV nodal pathway region, typically has those AV nodal pathways with the shortest refractory period that support the highest conduction frequencies. Ablation here may slow the ventricular response rate to AF without producing complete AV block. Nevertheless, in practice, this approach is frequently either ineffective or produces inadvertent complete AV block and, even when successful, the ventricular response remains irregular. Accordingly, this form of the procedure is rarely performed.

AF patients should be referred for consideration of the ablate-and-pace approach to rate control when other approaches to AF symptom control have failed or have been discarded (Box 7.1). The ablate-and-pace approach is most commonly used in elderly patients who are unlikely to out-live their pacemaker. It is also used for patients with a

---

Box 7.1 When to refer for the ablate-and-pace approach to AF management

- Patients with AF-related symptoms the relief of which warrants the risks of the approach.
- Usually after other approaches to AF symptom control have failed or have been considered to be inappropriate.
- Most commonly used in elderly patients.
- Patients with a cardiac resynchronization pacing system in whom rapid ventricular response rates are inhibiting biventricular pacing.

cardiac resynchronization pacemaker in whom rapid ventricular response rates inhibit biventricular pacing.

7.3 **The atrial fibrillation trigger and/or substrate ablation approach**

For many patients with a propensity to AF, surgical or transcatheter ablation of the triggers and/or maintenance substrates for AF may prevent subsequent AF and thereby accomplish both ventricular rate control and atrial tachyarrhythmia rhythm control.

The first approach to AF trigger and/or substrate ablation was surgical. After a series of modifications the Maze procedure now involves a biatrial cut-and-sew lesion set that isolates the pulmonary veins and the posterior left atrium along with compartmentalization of the remaining atria in a fashion originally expected to leave atrial compartments of insufficient mass as to perpetuate multiple wavelet re-entry. Less commonly, alternatives to cut-and-sew, including radiofrequency, laser, microwave, or cryoablation lesion sets are used. With the recognition that triggers for AF often originate from myocardial sleeves in the proximal portion of pulmonary veins, surgical AF trigger ablation may simply isolate the pulmonary veins from the left atrium. Regardless of the surgical approach used, the left atrial appendage (LAA) is usually removed or over-sewn.

The initial transcatheter approach to AF trigger and/or substrate ablation placed radiofrequency lesion lines in both the right atrium and the left atrium (approached with an atrial transseptal puncture) mimicking the surgical Maze procedure. Simplification of the procedure focused on isolation of the pulmonary veins from the left atrium—pulmonary vein isolation. Additional lesions may be added, including isolation of other veins entering the right or left atrium, placement of a right atrial cavotricuspid isthmus line, placement of left atrial lines, and ablation of areas of complex fractionated atrial electrograms (CAFEs or CFAEs), sites with high-frequency atrial electrograms, sites representing atrial rotors, or atrial ganglionated plexi. The ancillary ablations are directed at the AF maintenance substrate and are often used in patients with persistent AF rather than paroxysmal AF.

In a minority of patients, another tachyarrhythmia may be the trigger for AF. When the triggering tachyarrhythmia has a highly successful and low-risk ablation procedure, such as typical atrial flutter or a paroxysmal supraventricular tachycardia, the triggering tachyarrhythmia may be targeted for ablation to prevent AF. Nevertheless, ablation of such triggering tachyarrhythmias will prevent subsequent AF in less than half of such patients.

The major advantage of surgical AF trigger and/or substrate ablation is that it may establish AF rhythm control when other approaches have failed. Of course, the major advantages of transcatheter AF trigger and/or substrate ablation are the opportunity to accomplish this goal without cardiac surgery and the repeatability of transcatheter ablation. The probability of AF cure with an AF trigger and/or substrate ablation is dependent on many factors and is favoured by younger age, absent structural heart disease, paroxysmal rather than persistent AF, smaller left atrial size, absent sleep apnoea, absent obesity, multiple procedures, more extensive lesion sets, surgical ablation, and greater operator experience. Since the procedure involves extensive atrial ablation that may itself be arrhythmogenic, AF recurrences in the first 3 months after the ablation are usually discounted (the blanking period). Thereafter, expected 9-month follow-up AF/atrial flutter/atrial tachycardia non-recurrence rates in patients with paroxysmal AF after transcatheter AF trigger and/or substrate ablation are approximately 60% in the absence of antiarrhythmic drug therapy after a single procedure, 70% in the absence of antiarrhythmic drug therapy after multiple procedures, and 80% including antiarrhythmic drug therapy after multiple procedures. The success rates are higher after direct surgical AF trigger and/or substrate ablation and are lower in patients followed for longer periods of time and for patients with persistent AF. Randomized trials suggest that AF trigger and/or substrate ablation is associated with better AF rhythm control, exercise tolerance, quality of life, and LV systolic function than are either antiarrhythmic drug therapy (particularly after failure of an antiarrhythmic drug) or the ablate-and-pace approach. Another possible, but unproven, benefit of AF trigger and or substrate ablation is that it may lessen the risk of thromboembolic events when successful. Although AF trigger and/or substrate ablation is not recommended for the sole purpose of discontinuing anticoagulation, patients who have done so seem to have a lower than expected risk of subsequent stroke.

The major disadvantage of AF trigger and/or substrate ablation is the risk of the ablation procedure(s). Surgical AF trigger and/or substrate ablation exposes the patient to the risks of open-chest cardiac surgery including a 1–3% risk of death. With the transcatheter approach, each procedure carries a risk of significant adverse events in the range of 3–5%. The more common adverse events are cardiac perforation and tamponade (~1%), thromboembolic events including stroke or transient ischaemic attack (~1%), damage to femoral artery/vein (~1%), and other, less common, adverse events including symptomatic pulmonary vein stenosis and phrenic nerve paralysis. Fatal events are rare (~0.1%) but can occur late as a consequence of an atrio-oesophageal fistula (to be suspected when any post-ablation patient presents with haemodynamic compromise, unexplained fever, sepsis, or chest symptoms). On occasion, surgical or transcatheter AF trigger and/or substrate ablation may create even more bothersome atrial tachycardias or atrial flutters. The frequency of this complication is dependent upon the ablation technique used and may be as high as 15%. The other major disadvantage of transcatheter AF trigger and/or substrate ablation is its unimpressive success rate and the consequent likelihood of multiple procedures. Nevertheless, the success rates are higher than those of a single, or even multiple, class I or III antiarrhythmic drug trials.

AF patients should be referred for consideration of transcatheter AF trigger and/or substrate ablation when symptomatic after failure of one or more class I or III antiarrhythmic drugs when the potential advantages of the procedure(s) outweigh the risk of harm (Box 7.2). Many laboratories select patients for AF trigger and/or substrate ablation using characteristics suggesting a higher probability of enduring success and/or by the severity of the patient's AF symptoms. As the efficacy and safety of transcatheter AF trigger and/or substrate ablation have improved, the position of this approach in the cascade of therapeutic alternatives for AF patients has advanced. Some practitioners now consider transcatheter AF trigger and/or substrate ablation to be a viable first approach to treatment of some AF patients. AF patients are considered for surgical AF trigger and/or substrate ablation

---

Box 7.2 When to refer for AF trigger and/or substrate ablation

- Patients with AF-related symptoms the relief of which warrants the risks of the approach.
- Usually after failure of the rate control approach and at least one class I or III antiarrhythmic drug for the rhythm control approach.
- Most commonly used in younger patients with paroxysmal AF and absent structural heart disease.
- The surgical approach is usually reserved for failure of the transcatheter approach or for those patients with another indication for open chest cardiac surgery.

when there is another indication for open-chest cardiac surgery or when relief of AF symptoms has not been achieved despite one or more transcatheter AF trigger and/or substrate ablation procedures in whom maintenance of sinus rhythm is highly desired.

7.4 Device-based rhythm control approaches

A large number of other non-pharmacological approaches have been evaluated for their capacity to prevent or to rapidly terminate AF. These include atrial pacing in patients with a bradyarrhythmia indication for pacing, atrial pacing in patients without a brady-arrhythmia indication for pacing, alternative-site atrial pacing (Bachmann's bundle or interatrial septal pacing), multiple-site atrial pacing (dual right atrial or biatrial pacing), use of pacing algorithms to prevent AF initiation, use of pacing algorithms to terminate atrial tachyarrhythmias at the onset of AF, and use of the implantable atrial cardioverter. The rationales for these approaches to AF management include shortening atrial refractoriness, reducing spatial dispersion of atrial refractoriness, shorting atrial activation time, regularizing the ventricular response, reducing the frequency of atrial premature beats, and early termination of atrial tachyarrhythmias to prevent atrial remodelling that favours AF recurrences.

The theoretical advantages of device approaches to AF prevention and/or termination have not been realized with the exception of atrial-based pacing in patients with a bradyarrhythmia indication for pacing. Pacing may also be used to permit antiarrhythmic drug therapy for either AF rhythm control or ventricular response rate control without the bradyarrhythmia consequences of such therapy. Implanted devices have the advantage of providing rhythm monitoring data including that related to both atrial and ventricular arrhythmia episode rates, frequencies, durations, and timings. For some patients this advantage has been sufficient as to encourage development of stand-alone implantable devices to serve this purpose. The major disadvantages of device approaches to AF prevention and/or termination relate to the surgical and follow-up complications of an implanted device, atrial and/or ventricular proarrhythmia, and aggravation of LV systolic dysfunction secondary to pacing-induced ventricular dyssynchrony. The use of AF defibrillation devices has been limited by the inability to lower the defibrillation thresholds below that associated with shock therapy pain. Nevertheless, the possibility of device-based AF prevention and/or termination is still under investigation.

AF patients should be referred for consideration of device-based approaches to AF rhythm control when there is an independent indication for placement of a permanent cardiac rhythm control device—a bradyarrhythmia indication for a permanent pacemaker, a heart failure indication for a cardiac resynchronization pacing device, or a risk of ventricular tachyarrhythmia indication for an implantable defibrillator (Box 7.3).

Box 7.3 When to refer for implantable device therapy for AF prevention and/or termination

- Patients with AF-related symptoms the relief of which warrants the risks of the approach.
- Usually when there is an independent indication for placement of a permanent pacemaker.
- Often in order to preclude bradyarrhythmia responses to rate control or rhythm control antiarrhythmic drugs.

7.5 **Transcatheter left atrial appendage occlusion approaches**

In patients with AF, the most common source for the clot formation that predisposes to stroke or peripheral thromboembolism is the LAA. Thrombosis within the LAA may be responsible for 90% of thromboembolic events in this setting. Accordingly, mechanisms to exclude the LAA from the circulation have been sought. Over-sewing or excising the LAA at the time of cardiac surgery has been associated with reduction in subsequent thromboembolism risk. More recently, transcatheter approaches to LAA exclusion have been reported with the WATCHMAN device (Boston Scientific), the Amplatzer cardiac plug (St Jude Medical), the WaveCrest LAA occluder (Coherex Medical), and the Lariat LAA closure system (SentreHEART). The first three devices are placed after an atrial transseptal puncture; the last device requires both atrial transseptal access to the left atrium and access to the pericardial space in the manner of a pericardiocentesis. Of these systems, the WATCHMAN device has been most studied (Figure 7.1). Placement of the WATCHMAN device is usually followed by approximately 1.5 months of adjusted-dose warfarin (target international normalized ratio of 2.0–3.0). Thereafter, if transoesophageal echocardiography shows the device to be well seated without leaks, warfarin therapy is replaced by acetylsalicylic acid (ASA)/clopidogrel therapy for an additional 4.5 months followed by ASA therapy alone. Comparative clinical trials have suggested that this WATCHMAN strategy is at least non-inferior to adjusted-dose warfarin therapy alone and may be superior to warfarin in patients in whom the WATCHMAN device is successfully deployed.

The major advantage of transcatheter LAA closure is that it provides a means to prevent thromboembolic events including stroke that does not require either long-term oral anticoagulation or open-chest surgery.

The major disadvantages of current LAA occlusion devices are the inability to place the device in 2–5% of patients and a 2–10% probability of serious procedural complications such as cardiac tamponade, pericarditis, vascular injury, air embolism, device embolization, and thromboembolic events including stroke. The optimal strategy for anticoagulation and/or antiplatelet therapy after LAA occlusion device placement remains unknown. Short-term oral anticoagulation after device placement has been recommended for the WATCHMAN device and for the Amplatzer cardiac plug. Nevertheless, some procedures have been followed with antiplatelet therapy alone and a few have been followed by no anticoagulation or antiplatelet therapy. Comparative trials are not yet available. Finally, the risk of device infection over long-term follow-up remains to be established.

AF patients should be referred for consideration of transcatheter LAA closure when there are significant contraindications to oral anticoagulation (usually intractable bleeding events) despite a high $CHADS_2$ or CHA_2DS_2-VASc score in the absence of an absolute contraindication for oral anticoagulation as short-term anticoagulation is still required (Box 7.4). AF patients should also be considered for transcatheter LAA closure in combination with oral anticoagulation if thromboembolic events occur despite optimal oral

---

Box 7.4 When to refer for left atrial occlusion therapy

- AF patients at high risk of thromboembolic events for whom oral anticoagulation therapy is relatively or absolutely contraindicated.
- Usually such patients have had intractable bleeding events and do not have other evident sources of thrombus origin.
- AF patients with thromboembolic events despite optimal oral anticoagulation.

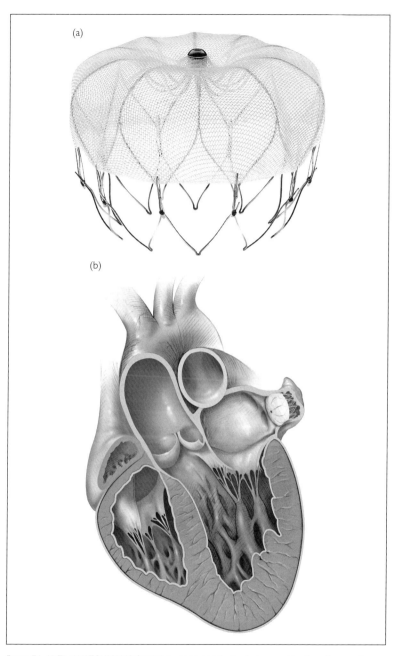

Figure 7.1 (a) The WATCHMAN left atrial appendage occlusion device consists of a self-expanding nitinol frame with fixation barbs covered by a permeable polyester fabric. (b) The Watchman device positioned in the left atrial appendage after having been delivered there by a transseptal catheter-based approach. © 2013 Boston Scientific Corporation or its affiliates. All rights reserved. Used with permission of Boston Scientific Corporation.

anticoagulation. The presence of sources of thromboembolism other than the LAA has been considered to identify patients unsuitable for LAA device closure therapy. Such alternative sources include an atrial septal defect, a patent foramen ovale with atrial septal aneurysm, a mechanical prosthetic heart valve, marked LV systolic dysfunction, complex aortic atheroma, and significant carotid artery disease.

Key reading

Anter E, Callans DJ. Surgical atrial fibrillation ablation: an electrophysiologist's perspective. *Card Electrophysiol Clin* 2012; 4: 395–402.

Betts TR. Atrioventricular junction ablation and pacemaker implant for atrial fibrillation: still a valid treatment in appropriately patients. *Europace* 2008; 10: 325–32.

Calkins H. Catheter ablation to maintain sinus rhythm. *Circulation* 2013; 125: 1439–45.

Calkins H, Kuck KH, Cappato R, Brugada J, Camm AJ, Chen S-A, *et al.* 2012 HRS/EHRA/ECAS expert consensus statement on catheter ablation and surgical ablation of atrial fibrillation: recommendations for patient selection, procedural techniques, patient management and follow-up, definitions, endpoints, and research trial design. *Heart Rhythm* 2012; 9: 632–96.

Horton RP, Doshi SK, Sánchez JE, Di Biase L, Natale A. Percutaneous closure of the left atrial appendage. *Card Electrophysiol Clin* 2012; 4: 383–94.

Knight BP, Gersh BJ, Carlson MD, Friedman PA, McNamara RL, Strickberger A, *et al.* Role of permanent pacing to prevent atrial fibrillation. *Circulation* 2005; 111: 240–3.

Leal S, Moreno R, de Sousa Almeida M, Silva JA, López-Sendón JL. Evidence-based percutaneous closure of the left atrial appendage in patients with atrial fibrillation. *Curr Cardiol Rev* 2012; 8: 37–42.

Lewalter T, Ibrahim R, Albers B, Camm AJ. An update and current expert opinions on percutaneous left atrial appendage occlusion for stroke prevention in atrial fibrillation. *Europace* 2013; 15: 652–6.

Silberbauer J, Sulke N. The role of pacing in rhythm control and management of atrial fibrillation. *J Interv Card Electrophysiol* 2007; 18: 159–86.

Thomas SP, Sanders P. Catheter ablation for atrial fibrillation. *Heart Lung Circ* 2012; 21: 395–401.

Wann LS, Curtis AB, Ellenbogen KA, Estes III NAM, Ezekowitz MD, Jackman WM, *et al.* 2011 ACCF/AHA/HRS focused updates incorporated into the ACC/AHA/ESC 2006 guidelines for the management of patients with atrial fibrillation. *J Am Coll Cardiol* 2011; 57:e101–98.

Chapter 8

Summary guidelines for the management of atrial fibrillation

Cevher Ozcan and Anne B. Curtis

> ### Key points
>
> - Effective management of atrial fibrillation (AF) is important for the prevention of AF-related morbidity and mortality. Practice guidelines provide specific recommendations for each aspect of management in order to provide optimal care to patients.
> - Prevention of thromboembolic events is essential in the management of AF regardless of treatment strategy (rate versus rhythm control). The patient's risk score (CHA_2DS_2-VASc) should be assessed and anticoagulation prescribed as indicated by guideline recommendations.
> - Rate control is indicated in patients with permanent AF, and it is a reasonable first-line strategy in elderly patients with minimally symptomatic AF. A resting heart rate lower than 80 beats per minute should be the goal in most patients with AF.
> - Maintenance of sinus rhythm should be considered in patients with new-onset AF or early in the course of paroxysmal and persistent AF. When severe electrical and structural remodelling occurs, sinus rhythm may be more difficult to restore or maintain.
> - Antiarrhythmic drugs are the first choice in most cases to maintain sinus rhythm, but catheter ablation is a viable option in many patients if antiarrhythmic drugs are ineffective or not tolerated.

8.1 Guidelines and management of atrial fibrillation

The management of atrial fibrillation (AF) has evolved substantially in the past decade as a result of new therapeutic options and novel strategies. Clinical practice guidelines provide recommendations for the management of patients with AF based on clinical studies, evolving data, and expert opinion. The recommendations are developed to improve patient outcomes and quality of care with evidence-based practice.

Appropriate management of AF is important to minimize morbidity and mortality related to AF. The practice guidelines for AF mainly focus on three areas: prevention of thromboembolic events, rate control, and rhythm control (Figure 8.1). Recently, there have been several major updates to the guidelines for the management of AF, including antiplatelet and anticoagulant therapy, new antithrombotic agents, recommendations on heart rate control, new antiarrhythmic agents, as well as non-pharmacological rhythm control strategies. In

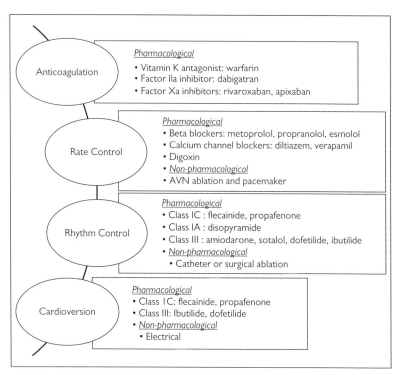

Figure 8.1 Summary of options for the management of atrial fibrillation: anticoagulation therapy, heart rate control, rhythm control, and cardioversion. Class IC, IA and III are as cited in the Vaughan Williams Classification of Antiarrhythmic Drugs. AVN = atrioventricular node.

this chapter, we summarize the fundamental points of the current practice guidelines of the American College of Cardiology (ACC), American Heart Association (AHA), and Heart Rhythm Society (HRS) for the management of patients with AF. Our goal is to simplify the recommendations for practitioners to apply the guidelines in their practice to provide the optimal standard of care to patients with AF.

8.2 **Prevention of thromboembolic events in atrial fibrillation**

Thromboembolic events are a major cause of morbidity and mortality in patients with AF. Prevention of thromboembolic events is essential in the management of AF regardless of the chosen treatment strategy, rate versus rhythm control. Once a patient has been identified as having AF, the decision about whether and how to anticoagulate the patient should be based on the patient's risk factors for thromboembolism and not the type or frequency of AF. The reason for this recommendation is that paroxysmal AF carries approximately the same risk of thromboembolic events as persistent or permanent AF. The only exception to this rule of thumb may be the occasional patient who has demonstrated a single episode of AF under extreme circumstances (e.g. hospitalization for pneumonia). In such cases, whether a patient should receive long-term prophylaxis against stroke should be determined based on the likelihood of further episodes of AF (electrocardiographic (ECG) monitoring in the outpatient setting may be helpful in decision-making) and the patient's risk for thromboembolic events.

There are two risk scores that have been used in patients with AF (Table 8.1). The $CHADS_2$ schema identifies heart failure, hypertension, age 75 years or above, diabetes mellitus (1 point for each), and previous stroke or transient ischaemic attack (2 points) as risk factors for stroke. More recently, the CHA_2DS_2-VASc score has been introduced, which has two age categories (65–74 years (1 point) and >75 years (2 points)) and also adds female sex and vascular disease as additional risk factors (1 point each). The CHA_2DS_2-VASc score is now recommended for assessment of stroke risk in patients with non-valvular AF by the latest AHA/ACC/HRS guideline. Any CHA_2DS_2-VASc patient with a score of 2 or higher should receive anticoagulation. Patients with a CHA_2DS-VASc score of 0 do not require anticoagulation. Those with a score of 1 can be treated with aspirin, an oral anticoagulant, or no therapy; in such cases, the decision should be made based on the component of the CHA_2DS_2-VASc score that is positive and the tolerance of the patient for stroke versus the potential for bleeding.

There are also risk scores that have been developed to assess a patient's risk for bleeding. One such example is HAS-BLED (hypertension, abnormal liver or renal function, history of stroke, history of bleeding, history of labile international normalized ratios (INRs), elderly, and use of drugs or alcohol). Many of these risk factors are the same as those in CHA_2DS_2-VASc. Given that reality, only in select circumstances is the risk of bleeding likely to trump concerns about thromboembolic events and lead to a decision not to anticoagulate a patient at a high risk of stroke.

Current guidelines recommend pharmacological prevention of thromboembolism with anticoagulation. Non-pharmacological options such as left atrial appendage (LAA) occlusion devices are still under investigation at the present time, and therefore no specific recommendations have been made yet in the practice guidelines. However, surgical excision of the LAA may be considered in patients undergoing cardiac surgery.

Table 8.1 Anticoagulation strategy based on risk score in patients with atrial fibrillation

CHA_2DS_2-VASc score	Treatment options for anticoagulation
0	No anticoagulation
1	No anticoagulation, or aspirin, warfarin, dabigatran, rivaroxaban, or apixaban
≥ 2	Warfarin, dabigatran, rivaroxaban, or apixaban

CHA_2DS_2-VASc identifies heart failure, hypertension, diabetes mellitus, vascular disease, female sex (1 point for each), and previous stroke or transient ischaemic attack (2 points). Also, it has two age categories: 65–74 years (1 point) and ≥ 75 years (2 points).

Reproduced from *Heart Rhythm*, 9:4, Calkins et al., 2012 HRS/EHRA/ECAS Expert Consensus Statement on Catheter and Surgical Ablation of Atrial Fibrillations, 632–96, Copyright 2012, with permission from Elsevier.

Anticoagulation therapy for AF includes vitamin K antagonists, platelet inhibitors, and antithrombotic agents as discussed in Chapter 6. Current guidelines indicate that warfarin, dabigatran, rivaroxaban, or apixaban should be prescribed for patients with more than one moderate risk factor. Treatment with warfarin requires routine blood testing with adjustment of the dose to achieve a target INR of 2.0–3.0. Aspirin (81–325 mg daily) may be prescribed for low-risk patients. It is recognized that lone AF in younger (< 60 years) patients carries a low risk of thromboembolism, and long-term anticoagulation with a vitamin K antagonist is not indicated. For patients with one of the less well-validated risk factors, aspirin, an oral anticoagulant, or no therapy is reasonable for prevention of thromboembolism.

Given the availability of several new oral anticoagulants with efficacy comparable to that of warfarin, the combination of aspirin with clopidogrel is no longer recommended for thromboprophylaxis against stroke. However, clopidogrel may be used in combination with an anticoagulant, but without aspirin, after coronary revascularization.

In addition to dabigatran, a direct thrombin inhibitor, two factor Xa inhibitors (rivaroxaban and apixaban) have recently been introduced into clinical practice as novel oral anticoagulants for AF. The latest guideline states that all three drugs have a Class 1 recommendation for anticoagulation in AF. Dabigatran, rivaroxaban, and apixaban are acceptable alternatives to warfarin for the prevention of stroke and systemic thromboembolism in patients with paroxysmal to permanent AF who do not have a prosthetic heart valve or significant valve disease.

The choice of an anticoagulant should take into consideration the patient's clinical condition. For example, patients with significant renal disease should be treated with warfarin, as the other available agents are renally excreted. Another consideration is compliance. Warfarin requires blood test monitoring and dose adjustment, and failure to maintain a therapeutic INR means loss of protection against thromboembolism. On the other hand, abrupt discontinuation of one of the newer anticoagulants such as rivaroxaban has been shown to be associated with a higher risk of thromboembolic events. One other factor to consider is the lack of a specific reversal agent with the newer anticoagulants, if serious bleeding occurs.

For most patients, it is reasonable to interrupt anticoagulation for up to 1 week for procedures that carry a risk of bleeding. For high-risk patients (e.g. recent stroke), continuation of anticoagulation or bridging with heparin may be necessary.

8.3 **Rate control in atrial fibrillation**

Ventricular rate control is commonly used for patients with AF. It is important to control the ventricular rate in order to improve a patient's haemodynamics, symptoms, and quality of life. Effective rate control facilitates adequate time for ventricular filling and precludes tachycardia-induced ischaemia and cardiomyopathy. Indeed, tachycardia-related cardiomyopathy is reversible by controlling the ventricular rate.

With new-onset AF, rate control is commonly attempted first, followed by restoration of sinus rhythm if appropriate. However, if a patient develops symptomatic hypotension, angina, or heart failure, prompt cardioversion will be necessary.

In addition to anticoagulation, rate control is a first-line treatment recommendation for patients with permanent AF. It is also a reasonable strategy in elderly patients with minimally symptomatic AF. Rate control is usually a short-term treatment goal in symptomatic patients with paroxysmal and persistent AF until a rhythm control strategy is implemented.

The target ventricular rate for effective rate control should be determined based on an individual patient's co-morbidities, clinical characteristics, and functional need. The efficacy of rate control should be evaluated during rest and exercise. Current practice guidelines suggest that a heart rate control (resting heart rate < 80 beats per minute (bpm)) strategy is reasonable for symptomatic management of AF. A more lenient rate control strategy (<110 bpm at rest) may be reasonable in selected patients if they are asymptomatic and left ventricular systolic function is preserved.

Rate control can be achieved with pharmacological and non-pharmacological approaches, including atrioventricular (AV) nodal blocking medications or AV junction ablation and pacing. Pharmacological rate control is always the first-line treatment, but AV junction ablation with permanent pacemaker implantation is an alternative approach if medications fail to control the rate and catheter ablation of AF has failed or is not an option. In such cases, particularly if there is any component of heart failure, cardiac resynchronization therapy is often considered as the modality for pacing.

There are several drugs that are used for pharmacological rate control, particularly beta blockers and the non-dihydropyridine calcium channel antagonists (verapamil and diltiazem). These agents may be given intravenously in the acute setting, or there are oral formulations for long-term management. Careful dose adjustment is required to achieve optimal rate control and also to prevent symptomatic bradycardia and heart block. Intravenous amiodarone is an effective rate control agent in the acute setting if other drugs have failed to control the ventricular rate or are contraindicated.

Selection of an AV nodal blocking agent should be individualized based on a patient's underlying characteristics. Beta blockers should be the first-line agents for most patients for rate control. If adequate rate control is not achieved or sufficient doses of the drug are not tolerated, then other drugs such as diltiazem, verapamil, or digoxin can be added. Digoxin is often suggested for patients with heart failure or left ventricular dysfunction, or for those who have a sedentary lifestyle. Digoxin should not be used as the sole rate control agent in patients with paroxysmal AF to control the rate at rest and during exercise, but rather it should be combined with a beta blocker or a calcium channel antagonist. Calcium channel antagonists are not recommended in patients with decompensated heart failure since they can cause haemodynamic compromise.

For rapid control of the ventricular rate in AF, an intravenous beta blocker or diltiazem is usually given. Digoxin may be added if necessary to achieve adequate rate control. Intravenous digoxin or calcium channel antagonists may paradoxically accelerate the ventricular response to AF in patients with pre-excitation syndromes (e.g. Wolff–Parkinson–White syndrome). If such a patient is haemodynamically stable, intravenous procainamide or amiodarone is recommended in the acute setting.

Non-pharmacological therapy should be considered when pharmacological measures fail or cause significant side effects. However, with the increasing use of catheter ablation for the cure of AF, it should be noted that fewer patients undergo AV junction ablation and permanent pacemaker implantation than in the past, because of the pacemaker dependency that results and the lack of effect on the primary substrate. Good candidates for AV junction ablation may include, for example, those who have failed multiple ablation procedures, those who have contraindications to or who are unwilling to undergo primary ablation for AF, or those who are elderly and have minimal symptoms except for those due to elevated heart rates. It should be noted that some patients may simply need permanent pacemaker implantation to protect against drug-induced bradycardia, and then AV nodal blocking drugs may control the ventricular rate without the need for AV junction ablation.

AV junction ablation in conjunction with permanent pacemaker implantation is highly effective in controlling the heart rate. It improves symptoms, quality of life, left ventricular function, exercise capacity, and healthcare utilization for patients with symptomatic, drug-refractory AF. This strategy has no negative impact on long-term survival compare to rhythm control. However, chronic right ventricular apical pacing after AV junction ablation may lead to adverse ventricular remodelling and heart failure over time. Therefore, biventricular pacing should be considered in patients with a left ventricular ejection fraction of 50% or lower, as a recent study showed that patients with AV block and an ejection fraction as high as 50% benefit from biventricular pacing compared to right ventricular pacing with respect to clinical outcomes and ventricular remodelling.

8.4 **Rhythm control in AF**

Restoring and maintaining sinus rhythm is the optimal long-term therapeutic goal for the majority of patients with AF. Sinus rhythm is physiological and maintains the atrial contribution to left ventricular filling. A rhythm control strategy prevents atrial electrical and structural remodelling related to AF and therefore delays progression of the disease process. Maintaining sinus rhythm in paroxysmal AF may inhibit the development of persistent and permanent AF. Rhythm control should be considered in patients with new-onset AF or early in the course of paroxysmal and persistent AF. Sinus rhythm may not be restored or maintained once severe electrical and structural remodelling develops.

Restoration and maintenance of sinus rhythm can be achieved pharmacologically with antiarrhythmic drugs and non-pharmacologically with catheter ablation. Before initiating a rhythm control strategy, it is essential to treat precipitating or reversible causes of AF. Then, pharmacological or electrical cardioversion may be required to restore sinus rhythm in patients with AF while starting a rhythm control strategy. In current practice, antiarrhythmic drugs are the first-line treatment for rhythm control. If antiarrhythmic drugs fail to control the arrhythmia or are not tolerated, catheter ablation may be offered to appropriate patients. In selected cases, catheter ablation may be considered as first-line treatment for AF. Simplified guideline recommendations for antiarrhythmic drugs and catheter ablation for rhythm control in AF are presented in Figure 8.2.

Antiarrhythmic drugs are commonly used for the long-term management of patients with AF. Class III (amiodarone, sotalol, dofetilide, ibutilide, dronedarone) and class IC (flecainide and propafenone) antiarrhythmic drugs are the main choices for maintaining and restoring sinus rhythm as discussed in Chapter 5. Selection of an antiarrhythmic drug is based on a patient's clinical characteristics (Figure 8.2). Class IC agents are recommended for patients without structural heart disease. They are generally well tolerated, and they have a low incidence of extra-cardiac side effects. They are usually given in conjunction with an AV nodal blocking agent. Class III agents are appropriate for patients with underlying cardiovascular disease. For patients with heart failure, either amiodarone or dofetilide are reasonable choices to maintain sinus rhythm. On the other hand, sotalol and dronedarone should be avoided in patients with heart failure. Overall, antiarrhythmic drugs are moderately effective in maintaining sinus rhythm. The efficacy of antiarrhythmic drugs is fairly comparable except for amiodarone, which has been shown to be more effective than other antiarrhythmics in maintaining sinus rhythm and preventing recurrences of AF.

Antiarrhythmic drugs may be proarrhythmic and may be associated with other side effects. Certain antiarrhythmic drugs with predominantly class III effects (dofetilide, sotalol) may cause QT prolongation and torsades de pointes. Thus, these drugs should be started in a hospital setting while monitoring the electrocardiogram closely for QT interval prolongation. This approach is required when starting dofetilide, and is recommended in many cases when starting sotalol. One other caution is that pharmacological rhythm control agents should not be used in patients with significant sinus node or AV nodal conduction disease if the patient does not have a permanent pacemaker.

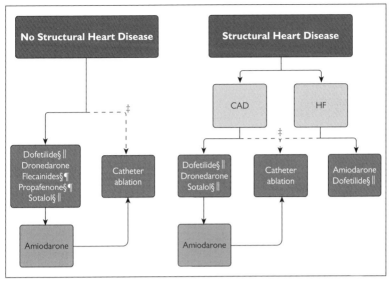

Figure 8.2 The management of patients with recurrent paroxysmal or persistent atrial fibrillation based on the recommendations of the ACCF/AHA/HRS 2014 guideline.

*Catheter ablation is only recommended as first-line therapy for patients with paroxysmal AF (Class IIa recommendation).

†Drugs are listed alphabetically.

‡Depending on patient preference when performed in experienced centers.

§Not recommended with severe LVH (wall thickness >1.5 cm).

‖Should be used with caution in patients at risk for torsades de pointes ventricular tachycardia.

¶Should be combined with AV nodal blocking agents.

AF = atrial fibrillation; CAD =coronary artery disease; HF = heart failure; LVH = left ventricular hypertrophy.

From January CT, Wann LS, Alpert JS, Calkins H, Cleveland JC Jr, Cigarroa JE, et al. 2014 AHA/ACC/ HRS guideline for the management of patients with atrial fibrillation: A report of the American College of Cardiology/American Heart Association Task Force on practice guidelines and the Heart Rhythm Society. Circulation Published online before print March 28, 2014.

The latest guidelines for the management of AF state that 'AF catheter ablation is useful for symptomatic paroxysmal AF refractory or intolerant to at least 1 class I or III antiarrhythmic medication when a rhythm control strategy is desired'. Indeed, in the past decade, there have been substantial advances in catheter ablation techniques and the rate of procedural success. Catheter ablation of AF must be performed by an experienced practitioner with optimal technique. The procedure-related complication rate has been reduced with standardization of the technique and increased experience. As a result, catheter ablation for AF is now recommended as a reasonable alternative to drug therapy for restoring and maintaining sinus rhythm. The long-term outcome for maintaining sinus rhythm with catheter ablation is superior to that with antiarrhythmic drugs in patients with paroxysmal AF. The success rate with catheter ablation is higher for paroxysmal AF than it is for persistent or long-standing persistent AF. Catheter ablation may now also be considered as a first-line treatment for paroxysmal AF in selected patients. Indications for catheter ablation of AF

Table 8.2 Recommendations for catheter ablation of atrial fibrillation based on the 2014 AHA/ACC/HRS guideline

Indications for catheter ablation of atrial fibrillation (AF)	Class	Level of evidence
Symptomatic AF refractory or intolerant to at least one class 1 or 3 antiarrhythmic medication		
Paroxysmal: catheter ablation is recommended	I	A
Persistent: catheter ablation is reasonable	IIa	A
Longstanding persistent: catheter ablation may be considered	IIb	B
Symptomatic AF prior to initiation of antiarrhythmic drug therapy with a class 1 or 3 antiarrhythmic agent		
Paroxysmal: catheter ablation is reasonable	IIa	B
Persistent: catheter ablation may be considered	IIb	C
Longstanding persistent: catheter ablation may be considered	IIb	C

Catheter ablation is a reasonable alternative to pharmacological therapy in symptomatic patients with AF. It is associated with a lower success rate or a higher complication rate in the presence of concomitant heart disease, obesity/sleep apnoea, large left atrial size, left ventricular dysfunction, and longer duration of continuous AF.

From January CT, Wann LS, Alpert JS, Calkins H, Cleveland JC Jr, Cigarroa JE, et al. 2014 AHA/ACC/HRS guideline for the management of patients with atrial fibrillation: A report of the American College of Cardiology/American Heart Association Task Force on practice guidelines and the Heart Rhythm Society. Circulation Published online before print March 28, 2014.

are summarized in Table 8.2 based on the latest recommendations in the guideline. The latest guideline also states that an AF surgical ablation procedure (Maze) is reasonable for selected patients with AF undergoing cardiac surgery for other indication.

8.5 **Cardioversion**

Cardioversion may be required immediately in an acute setting or performed electively to restore sinus rhythm in patients with persistent AF. The practice guidelines recommend pharmacological or non-pharmacological cardioversion based on a patient's condition. In general, cardioversion is performed in the hospital with close haemodynamic monitoring. If AF has been present for less than 48 hours, one may proceed with cardioversion immediately, along with initiation of anticoagulation. If AF has been present for more than 48 hours, or if the duration is unknown, then a patient should be anticoagulated appropriately for at least 3 weeks before elective cardioversion. An alternative approach is to perform a transoesophageal echocardiogram. If no thrombus is seen in the left atrium, then cardioversion may be performed immediately, as long as anticoagulation is instituted as well. It should be noted that there is no difference between pharmacological and electrical methods of cardioversion with respect to the risk of thromboembolism or stroke.

Current guidelines recommend administration of flecainide, dofetilide, propafenone, or ibutilide as first-line agents for pharmacological cardioversion of AF. An attractive option for chemical cardioversion in patients without structural heart disease is the administration of one of the class 1C antiarrhythmic drugs, flecainide or propafenone. This 'pill-in-the-pocket' approach is highly effective and can be used outside the hospital for converting

AF to sinus rhythm with a single oral dose, although it is recommended that the patient be monitored the first time this approach is used.

Intravenous administration of ibutilide is more effective than the other drugs in restoring sinus rhythm. In addition to flecainide or propafenone, dofetilide is modestly successful in converting AF to sinus rhythm. Amiodarone is also a reasonable option for cardioversion, but its effect is delayed. Sotalol is not effective for cardioversion. There are not enough data on the utility of quinidine, disopyramide, or procainamide for cardioversion, although these drugs are rarely used today. Pharmacological cardioversion carries the risk of drug-induced torsades de pointes or other serious arrhythmias. Moreover, it is less effective than electrical cardioversion. However, pharmacological cardioversion has the advantage of not requiring conscious sedation or anaesthesia. Pharmacological cardioversion is most effective within 7 days of the onset of an AF episode.

Direct-current electrical energy is used for non-pharmacological cardioversion. Delivery of an electric shock (usually biphasic) is synchronized with the patient's intrinsic rhythm by sensing the R wave of the electrocardiogram. Electrical cardioversion is more effective than pharmacological cardioversion, but it requires conscious sedation or anaesthesia during the procedure. There is an absolute indication for immediate electrical cardioversion if AF causes acute heart failure, hypotension, or worsening of angina pectoris. Also, electrical cardioversion is recommended in patients with pre-excitation in AF. Electrical cardioversion is not recommended in the setting of hypokalaemia and digitalis toxicity.

If needed, pretreatment with ibutilide may enhance the success of direct-current cardioversion. Antiarrhythmic drugs such as amiodarone, flecainide, propafenone, sotalol, dofetilide, or dronedarone may be started prior to electrical cardioversion to improve the chance of maintaining sinus rhythm after successful cardioversion.

8.6 Upstream therapies for prevention of atrial fibrillation

While some studies have shown beneficial effects of angiotensin-converting enzyme (ACE) inhibitors, angiotensin receptor antagonists (ARBs), and HMG CoA-reductase inhibitors (statins) in the primary and secondary prevention of AF, the results have not been consistent. Thus, the guidelines do not recommend the routine use of these drugs for the prevention of AF in patients without cardiovascular disease. However, the latest guidelines suggest that an ACE inhibitor or ARB is reasonable for primary prevention of new-onset AF in patients with HF with reduced left ventricular ejection fraction. Also, they may be considered for primary prevention of new-onset AF in the setting of hypertension. Statins may be reasonable for prevention of new-onset AF after coronary artery bypass surgery.

8.7 Conclusion

The management of AF has evolved significantly in the past few years, resulting in several major updates to the guidelines regarding anticoagulation and rate and rhythm control strategies. Anticoagulation to prevent thromboembolic events should be based on a patient's risk stratification. Pharmacological rate and rhythm control are the first-line recommendations for AF based on a patient's individual clinical characteristics. If pharmacological management fails or causes significant side effects, non-pharmacological interventions such as catheter ablation should be considered. The patient's management strategy should be evaluated and updated regularly to prevent morbidity and mortality in AF. Practice guidelines provide optimal recommendations for patient care in AF.

Key reading

Calkins H, Kuck KH, Cappato R, Brugada J, Camm AJ, Chen SA, et al. 2012 HRS/EHRA/ECAS expert consensus statement on catheter and surgical ablation of atrial fibrillation: recommendations for patient selection, procedural techniques, patient management and follow-up, definitions, endpoints, and research trial design. Heart Rhythm 2012; 9(4): 632–96.

Calkins H, Reynolds MR, Spector P, Sondhi M, Xu Y, Martin A, et al. Treatment of atrial fibrillation with antiarrhythmic drugs or radiofrequency ablation: two systematic literature reviews and meta-analyses. Circ Arrhythm Electrophysiol 2009; 2(4): 349–61.

Connolly S, Pogue J, Hart R, Pfeffer M, Hohnloser S, Chrolavicius S, Yusuf S. Clopidogrel plus aspirin versus oral anticoagulation for atrial fibrillation in the Atrial fibrillation Clopidogrel Trial with Irbesartan for prevention of Vascular Events (ACTIVE W): a randomised controlled trial. Lancet 2006; 367: 1903–12.

Connolly SJ, Ezekowitz MD, Yusuf S, Eikelboom J, Oldgren J, Parekh A, et al. Dabigatran versus warfarin in patients with atrial fibrillation. N Engl J Med 2009; 361: 1139–51.

Cosedis Nielsen J, Johannessen A, Raatikainen P, Hindricks G, Walfridsson H, Kongstad O, et al. Radiofrequency ablation as initial therapy in paroxysmal atrial fibrillation. N Engl J Med 2012; 367(17): 1587–95.

Curtis AB. Practice implications of the atrial fibrillation guidelines. Am J Cardiol 2013; 111(11): 1660–70.

Fuster V, Rydén LE, Cannom DS, Crijns HJ, Curtis AB, Ellenbogen KA, et al. 2011 ACCF/AHA/HRS focused updates incorporated into the ACC/AHA/ESC 2006 guidelines for the management of patients with atrial fibrillation. Circulation 2011; 123(10): e269–367.

Goldstein LB, Bushnell CD, Adams RJ, Appel LJ, Braun LT, Chaturvedi S, et al. Guidelines for the primary prevention of stroke: a guideline for healthcare professionals from the AHA/ASA. Stroke 2011; 42(2): 517–84.

January CT, Wann LS, Alpert JS, Calkins H, Cleveland JC Jr, Cigarroa JE, et al. 2014 AHA/ACC/HRS guideline for the management of patients with atrial fibrillation: A report of the American College of Cardiology/American Heart Association Task Force on practice guidelines and the Heart Rhythm Society. Circulation. Published online before print March 28, 2014.

Kirchhof P, Curtis AB, Skanes AC, Gillis AM, Wann SL, Camm JA. Atrial fibrillation guidelines across the Atlantic: a comparison of the current recommendations of the ESC/EHRS/EACS, the ACCF/AHA/HRS, and the CCS. Eur Heart J 2013; 34(20): 1471–4.

Ozcan C, Jahangir A, Friedman PA, Patel PJ, Munger TM, Rea RF, et al. Long-term survival after ablation of the atrioventricular node and implantation of a permanent pacemaker in patients with atrial fibrillation. N Engl J Med 2001; 344(14): 1043–51.

Smith MD, Crijns HJ, Tijssen JG, Hillege HL, Alings M, Tuininga YS, et al. Effect of lenient versus strict rate control on cardiac remodeling in patients with atrial fibrillation data of the RACE II. J Am Coll Cardiol 2011; 58(9): 942–9.

Wann LS, Curtis AB, January CT, Ellenbogen KA, Lowe JE, Estes NA 3rd, et al. 2011 ACCF/AHA/HRS focused update on the management of patients with atrial fibrillation (Updating the 2006 Guideline). Heart Rhythm 2011; 8(1): 157–76.

Weerasooriya R, Khairy P, Litalien J, Macle L, Hocini M, Sacher F, et al. Catheter ablation for atrial fibrillation: are results maintained at 5 years of follow-up? J Am Coll Cardiol 2011; 57(2): 160–6.

Wyse DG, Waldo AL, DiMarco JP, Domanski MJ, Rosenberg Y, Schron EB, et al. A comparison of rate control and rhythm control in patients with atrial fibrillation. N Engl J Med 2002; 347(23): 1825–33.

Index